"Our friend, Judy Seegmiller, takes us on a painful and realistic journey through the devastating stages of Alzheimer's. Judy triumphantly emerges with hope and promise stemming from her overwhelming faith and great love."

Dr. Stephen R. Covey, Author and Sandra Covey

"'Life with Big Al' has been the best book I have read to date on this subject, and I think I have read them all . . . In no other book or reference was I able to find such truth. I cried throughout most of the book . . . I was amazed at the similarities of our experiences. . . I feel like I have known Judy for years after reading the book."

Deb Carey, Caregiver

"Craig was the youngest person we had at The Alzheimer's Center. What I will always remember about Craig is his great love for Judy. He knew, to the end, who Judy was and that he was doing "good" if Judy was around. Her endless labor of love for Craig was an inspiration to all of us. What a tragedy to see someone in the prime of their existence to be struck by such a devastating disease. I hope that other caregivers will find reassurance that there are others out there like them through this book."

Marcia Lindelien, Director, The Alzheimer's Center

"This book is a painfully honest day-by-day account of a dedicated spouse dealing with her husband's fight with Alzheimer's disease. Alzheimer's not only created a child out of an otherwise healthy man, but it also deprived Judy of her best friend. Often one's contact with Alzheimer's patients consists of short visits or contacts in which the extent of the disease is not fully apparent. This book reveals the full impact of the disease on one's immediate family. True Christ-like service is required because the patient often not only isn't able to appreciate the efforts on his behalf, but also often greets those efforts with hostility and contempt. I will always remember how much small acts of kindness are appreciated by those struggling to cope with the changes in their lives brought about by the 'Big Al'."

Douglas A. Baxter, Attorney

"As an Emergency room physician I have seen many patients with Alzheimer's Disease. Not until I read Judy and Craig's diary, Life with Big Al, *did I more fully understand the burden it places on the caregivers. No one I know was more full of life, fun and enthusiasm than Craig. This is a story of love and tragedy. It was very hard for me to read. However, if you have a tough trail to hike in life this is the map you need to prepare for it."*

Keith R. Hooker, M.D., Alpine, UT

"As an Adult Protective Service worker, I do investigations on referrals of caregivers that are abusive, and neglectful towards their loved ones, or person(s) they are caring for with a disability. I have witnessed agonizing effects, and results of physical abuse, and validated the indignity of emotional and verbal abuse that has offended and shamed the disabled by their caregiver.

I was astounded by the paramount of strength Judy demonstrated not only mentally and physically but spiritually to preserve her husband's love and dignity throughout his devastating and deteriorating diseased course of Alzheimer's. Judy's diary, Life with Big Al, *will be a tool for other caregivers to assist them in learning skills through her experiences. Judy's diary teaches other families how they can pull together and alter their lifestyle in a positive manner by giving the disabled and the family a quality life during the deteriorating stages of the disease.*

Thank you Judy for writing your journal and sharing your experiences and knowledge that will inspire caregivers as they tread the difficult path of taking care of a loved one that has fallen victim to Alzheimer's and/or other forms of dementia."

Susan Orton, Adult Protective Services, Cedar City, UT

Life With
BIG AL
(Early Alzheimer's)

A Caregiver's Diary...

Judy Seegmiller

© 2000 Big Al. All rights reserved.
P.O. Box 50212
Provo, UT 84605-0212

No part of this publication may be reproduced, stored in a retrieval system, or transmitted in any form or by any means, electronic, photocopying, recording, or otherwise without the prior written permission of the publisher.

ISBN 1-57636-108-X

Printed in the United States of America

To the memory of my husband, Craig, a dear kind loving husband, father, grandfather & friend who made it to his graduation day touching us and redirecting our footsteps for good because of his great example.

ACKNOWLEDGMENT

Grateful acknowledgement to my wonderful children and their spouses: Steven and Wendy and Suzanne and Stephen and my grandchildren: Alex, Taylor, Emily, Madison, Jamison, Jordan and Maggie (who brought us such joy); Craig's wonderful friends (I feel so blessed to call them "our" friends); our store employees who are like family members; (they ran the store and kept it going those last years); and our family members. I am eternally grateful to them for being wonderful companions on this mission and walking this journey with me every step of the way. May you each be blessed.

A special thanks to Heather Frandsen for the cover design and formatting the book for print, to Robert Simpson for prodding me along and making the connections to make it all happen here locally, and to Jeff Alexander for believing in this project to print it and make it available to the public.

FOREWORD

I have never had the privilege of meeting Craig Seegmiller. The irony is, I didn't know of him at all until after he contracted early Alzheimer's disease and died way too early at the age of 55. It was then that his wife, Judy, sent me the manuscript for "Life with Big Al" and I got my crash course in the ecstasy and the agony that was Craig Seegmiller's life.

Judy's chronicle of the ordeal she shared with her husband touched me on two personal levels. First, I am of a similar vintage as Craig – barely five years younger. Second, my stepmother recently died of Alzheimer's disease.

So, the story hit home, as a Metro Columnist for the Deseret News in Salt Lake City, I was anxious to aid Judy in publicizing, through her "diary," the very personal side of a most insidious disease.

"Life with Big Al" caused me to reflect on the fragility of our human experience. No matter how invincible we might think we are, no matter how fit, how lean, how long we manage to dodge the flu, the fact is, we are most fortunate to be able to wake up every morning and to do it all again.

In truth, we're all tip-toeing through the minefield of life, dodging viruses, bacteria, falling rocks, fast cars, inorganic chemicals and most unavoidable of all, our own DNA.

If a man like Craig Seegmiller, a professional baseball player, a three-hour marathon runner, a man for whom a 10-mile run was a warm-down, can be taken in his prime, through absolutely no fault or cause of his own, what guarantees are there for the rest of us?

Where Judy's story touched me the most – and where I suspect it will have its most universal appeal – is in its descriptions of the realities of day-to-day coping with Alzheimer's. She applies a deft touch in communicating how such a devastating illness unavoidably alters the lives of all those affected. And how that altering can bring out the best, or the worst, in all of us.

As Craig walked inexorably into Alzheimer's purgatory, Judy walked right along with him, determined that the husband she adored and loved would not go anywhere abandoned and alone.

When my stepmother fell into the limbo netherworld of Alzheimer's, my sister, Karen made the same determination. For nearly seven long years Karen positioned herself at her mother's side, going where she went, doing what she did, propping her up the whole way.

I marveled that someone could be that dedicated, that loyal. Then after reading Judy Seegmiller's account, I marveled that two people could be that dedicated, that loyal. It is, as I see it, Alzheimer's only redeeming quality – that it allows others to shine brightly in contrast to its cruelly indifferent darkness.

"Life with Big Al" might seem to be a story about Alzheimer's disease. But it isn't that at all. Beyond the statistics and that "it could happen to anyone, anywhere" warning, it is above all a story about a man and a woman, and a family – a family that woke up one day and found Big Al had moved in.

When you finish reading, you'll love Judy and Craig and the rest of the family. And while you'll come to better understand Big Al, you'll also hate him. Getting rid of him should be no less than a crusade. In that way, Craig Seegmiller can keep on running.

Lee Benson, Columnist
Deseret News, Salt Lake City, UT

INTRODUCTION

I wrote about my (our) journey with 'Big Al' as a coping mechanism. My laptop was my therapist. It listened as I talked with my fingers on the keys…always listening and always there. It is my prayer that some of the words may help other Caregivers as they walk along this bumpy path that I walked. Our lives are so intertwined and how wonderful that we have the opportunity to reach out to others each day and they to us. My faith helped me tremendously. I belong to The Church of Jesus Christ of Latter-day Saints (Mormons). We believe not only in an afterlife – eternity; but that we will be an eternal family. Craig and I were sealed in the LDS temple for time and eternity. When you die you are buried in your temple attire which is sacred clothing you wear only inside the walls of the temple. I've learned to live one day at a time and with love in my heart and be ever so grateful for whatever that day may bring. Each day is a gift – a new dawning to be treasured. I learned that if I would take today, let yesterday go and not worry about tomorrow I could make it. I truly lived one day at a time. My children and I found that it was important to find the humor in 'Big Al' and to feel blessed that we had Craig for as long as we did. We felt it an honor and a privilege to care for him and fortunate that we had those 30 months to say "good-bye" each in our own way. We each approach death differently, arriving at the same destination with our own experiences, our own uniqueness. I hope that our journey, our map, will help someone in their journey to their destination or their loved one's destination.

Note: Craig called his disease, Early Alzheimer's, 'Big Al' after he was diagnosed.

AUTHOR'S NOTE

As you read the following pages I hope you realize that as hard as some of the days were I always felt a great deal of love and honor in caring for Craig. Even when I ached inside, cried my eyes out, prayed that he would shut his eyes and not wake up, and my words seemed to evoke sadness, I felt joy and happiness as I tried each day to "let my light shine." I also felt joy and happiness knowing that Craig's best interests were always uppermost in my thoughts and mind. I would do whatever it took each day to make everything right and good in his eyes. What an honor to serve and care for your soulmate the way I was able to serve and care for Craig. Not everyone has the opportunity I have had. I feel truly blessed because of this experience. My hope is that you will read these words and know that there is a great deal of joy to be found in service and great contentment in knowing that you gave it your all. You, as the Caregiver, need to be the one that strikes the match to dispel all the dark and you are the one that reminds others that a glass half empty is that same glass half full. It is okay to cry and feel sorrow but also remember to feel the joy. Our fortunes aren't in what we have but how we think, feel and care for those around us. Let others help you in your journey for they too will be blessed. I could not have done this alone. I believe our lives are intertwined and our thoughts and actions have ripple effects. How much richer we are because of each other. I had a thought that I read each day. It had no title and no author that I could find. It read: *"I asked God for strength that I might achieve, I was made weak that I might learn to obey. I asked for health that I might do greater things, I was given infirmity that I might do better things. I asked for riches that I might be happy. I was given poverty that I might be wise. I asked for power that I might have the praise of men, I was given weakness that I might feel the need of God. I asked for all things that I might enjoy life. I was given life that I might enjoy all things. I got nothing that I asked for — but everything I had hoped for. Almost despite myself, my unspoken prayers were answered. I am, among all men, most richly blessed."* I love thoughts and you will notice that even though my writing is sporadic I had a thought or a scripture for that day. I don't know where they came from but I've cherished in my heart the words for what seems forever.

To begin with, here is a little information about Alzheimer's. I give you this background before my story to help you understand the disease. Currently over 70 percent (2.7 million) of the 4 million Americans with the disease are cared for at home. They are cared for by spouses, relatives and friends. The incidence of home caregiving is expected to grow as an estimated 14 million Americans will develop the disease by the year 2050. Some 19 million Americans say a family member has the disease and 37 million Americans say they know someone with Alzheimer's. Half of all nursing home residents suffer from Alzheimer's disease or some other dementing illness. Doctors are getting better at diagnosing Alzheimer's based on clinical assessments. One of the reasons I think it is so important to try to correctly diagnose it is because there are different drugs that can help different kinds of dementia. So, if a person has Creutzfeldt-Jakob disease, Picks, etc. they could try different drugs to possibly help them rather than pigeonhole them to those found to help Alzheimer's.

The Alzheimer's Association gives 10 warning signals of Early Alzheimer's Disease.

(1) Recent memory loss that affects job skills. It's normal to forget people's names from time to time, but frequent forgetfulness is cause for concern.
(2) Difficulty performing familiar tasks. Anyone can leave a button unbuttoned. But when someone becomes persistently challenged by buttons, or other tasks of daily living most people take for granted, that's cause for concern.
(3) Language problems. From time to time, anyone can have difficulty finding the right word. But when simple words present problems, or when sentences become incomprehensible, that might signal Alzheimer's.

(4) Time and place disorientation. It's normal to forget the date or a destination. But people with Alzheimer's often feel lost standing across the street from their homes.
(5) Loss of judgment. Anyone can fail to notice that an item of clothing is stained. But when someone dresses completely inappropriately – wearing several shirts or mistaking underwear for a hat – that's cause for concern.
(6) Problems with abstract thinking. Anyone can struggle over balancing a checkbook. People with Alzheimer's forget what numbers are for and how to use them.
(7) Misplacing things. Anyone can misplace a wallet or keys. But when someone puts a wallet in the refrigerator or keys in the sink, that's cause for concern.
(8) Changes in mood or behavior. Changing moods are a fact of life. But people with Alzheimer's often exhibit rapid mood changes – from calm to tears to rage – for no apparent reason.
(9) Changes in personality. People often become more 'crotchety' as they become elderly. But Alzheimer's often makes people paranoid, very confused, or fearful.
(10) Loss of initiative. It's normal to get bored with daily activities. But when people lose much of their get-up-and-go, that's cause for concern.

It is still not clear whether the changes in brain tissue cause the disease, or whether they are the result of some other causative process. Most scientists believe that tangles and plaques are causative. As these brain cells stop working, part of the brain dies. Neurofibrillary tangles and senile plaques develop only in the parts of the brain that control memory and retention of learned information. Functions such as heartbeat, breathing and digestion remain unaffected. As a result, many people with severe Alzheimer's are otherwise healthy. Craig, as he declined, forgot how to walk, sit, eat and drink.

Clinical assessment typically begins with a doctor's consultation. A Sno, M. et al "A Standardized Technique for Establishing Onset and Duration of Symptoms of Alzheimer's disease – Archives of Neurology". Next comes a complete medical history to see if the observed problems might be caused by something else: complete blood work to determine vitamin deficiencies and lead poisoning; blood chemistry to check for kidney failure and thyroid problems; tests for syphilis and HIV infections; a possible lumbar puncture to obtain cerebrospinal fluid, which can diagnose meningitis and encephalitis; an electroencephalogram to check for Creutzfeldt-Jakob disease; and a CT scan or MRI to look for brain tumors, stroke, and other dementing brain conditions. Also, there are types of dementia, which might be treatable. (It was after Craig's MRI that you could see the amount of atrophy on the right and left sides of his brain). After all of these, a doctor conducts a structured interview with the loved ones to assess the affected person's degree of cognitive deterioration. When I found out the diagnosis I could hardly respond I cried so much. I can't imagine the impact had I not realized before I was told. I did not take Craig with me where he could ever hear me talk to anyone about him and Alzheimer's. I remember when I made the appointment for the neurologist and they insisted I bring him if the appointment was for him. I had to make an appointment for myself in order to go by myself. When the neurologist talked to me and understood what I was doing he was kind enough not to charge me for my visit. Next, comes an interview with the affected individual to assess cognitive competence. Usually a Mini-Mental State Examination is given. It is a brief 11-question test developed in 1965 and asks a variety of questions—the year, season, date, day, month; the person's state, county, and town of residence; plus a list—repetition exercise, a serial subtraction exercise, and simple writing, copying, and task-completion exercises. The person gets points for correct answers and based on thousands of scores over 30 years of using this test, relative level of mental competence or dementia can be estimated. The medical doctor performed this test on Craig and he failed every question. He was so nervous. He kept looking at me for the answers. He cried when we left. I asked him why he was crying because he got every answer right, not wrong. He just misunderstood the doctor because I did the same thing last week. I knew we had to progress through further tests to determine without a shadow of doubt what we were dealing with. We then went through a Neuropsychological Evaluation with a clinical psychologist. He went through Craig's medical, psychiatric history, family background, academic, work history, test observations and mental status, speech/language functions, sensation/perception, visual-spatial/constructional ability, motor function, intellectual function and personality function. His writing was so deteriorated and he was so confused that I filled out all the forms. The tests showed markedly impaired function on overall neuropsychological ability with apparent dramatic loss in intellectual ability with only crystallized verbal intelligence being spared. Memory function was even more impacted though he still had good remote memory. The most primitive hand-eye coordination and visual-spatial processing had also been impacted. This is seen usually only in someone in the advanced stages of dementia of the Alzheimer's type. His intellectual functioning at this time had so diminished that on a Full Scale Weschler IQ his was 62. This was a nightmare for Craig and there are no words to describe the heartache I felt. Most people with Alzheimer's disease live for seven to ten years after diagnosis, and spend about five years under vigilant care either at home or in a nursing facility. Those with younger Alzheimer's usually deteriorate faster than an older person diagnosed with the disease. Alzheimer's disease is not considered fatal. Cause of death is quite varied: heart disease, stroke, various infections, etc. Craig ultimately died of kidney failure but it was due to Alzheimer's disease. It showed Alzheimer's on his death certificate and listed that as the cause of death in his obituary. I feel it very important to be honest and upfront so that people become aware of this terrible disease. It will never be out in the forefront if the disease is kept hidden and if we hide these individuals afflicted with the disease.

Fifty years ago, people with serious illnesses were often not told of their status for fear of upsetting them. More recently, the pendulum has swung the other way – toward full disclosure. I'm sure there are those that believe people have a right to know and to plan and prepare for their future. I believed I knew Craig's future and I wanted him to think it would be brighter than the one I knew it to be. So, I chose not to tell him the truth. There was a study done at a university with elderly people and they stated they would NOT want to be told of a diagnosis of Alzheimer's. I personally would not want to know because as I deteriorated I would not know it. This confirmed my decision not to tell Craig. Besides, his first comment was that he wanted to die. As we held each other he said, "You know Kevorkian isn't that bad." That thought frightened me and wanted to protect him even more from the truth. The diagnosis of Alzheimer's pushes loved ones to the edge. There is an all-consuming responsibility of caregiving that produce complex and contradictory responses within a family. Ours was no different. I did have the complete support of my children, which was the most important support system to me. It truly is a labor of love that is also frustrating, draining and very painful. Each person also deals with stress differently which complicates some relationships. It is important to try to work through the challenges as much as you can because otherwise the primary caregiver will burn out as the patient's disease progresses. Because of the reaction of some individuals around me I had to let a lot of things go and remind myself it was 'their' way of dealing with Alzheimer's. One of Craig's family members wanted a third opinion and one thought that he had been hit in the head as a youngster. You can't place blame. You can only feel sorrow. The person who has Alzheimer's is also their loved one and each person handles crisis in their own way. Craig, Steven, Suzanne and myself were already close. We've always been close and very supportive of each other. This brought us even closer as his caregivers. (Note that there are studies being done on children of Alzheimer's sufferers to yield clues to this disease.) His family helped in the beginning when we could take Craig to them. This is not easy and it takes a lot of planning and transitioning to allow everyone to adjust. As the disease progressed it was harder to take him to places. If you can arrange for help, do so. It became easier to leave him in familiar surroundings with as little disruption as possible. Having a loved one with Alzheimer's at home can prove distracting if you still work – I did. The people I worked for were great at allowing me flexibility. U.S. businesses lose billions of dollars in productivity and absenteeism. I used my vacation and sick days. Most businesses think they don't need to worry because this is an "old" person's disease. Productivity costs are even greater. Productivity as a general rule is estimated at up to twice your actual compensation. There are over 245,000 people a year under the age of 65 who get Alzheimer's, and many continue to work and make decisions until they suffer significant cognitive impairment.

Your home and familiar surroundings take on new meaning. There are changes in household dynamics in many ways. You rearrange your home to accommodate the new "child" you have living with you. We had one stair from the kitchen to our family room. This was very hard for Craig to navigate. Also, driving in a car is troublesome at getting them in and out. I had a doctor sign papers so that I could get a Handicapped plaque to hang in the window. This was a wonderful tool…extremely helpful.

Finances—it's expensive taking care of a person with Alzheimer's and as they deteriorate it gets even more expensive. We no longer had any income from Craig. All the money the store made went back into the store to pay employees, etc. Owning a small business we should have made a plan. You spend time building equity but that equity disappears when the key person is gone. (There was an article written in the March 8th edition of The Salt Lake Tribune using our store as an example) It is estimated that Alzheimer's disease costs the United States some $95 billion a year in lost productivity, medical care and personal caretakeing. For Alzheimer's sufferers cared for at home, the average out-of-pocket cost to family caregivers (excluding lost wages) is $12,500 per year. For Alzheimer's sufferers in nursing homes, average cost is $42,000 per year per person. The average cost of an Alzheimer's sufferer's care from diagnosis until death is $174,000, making Alzheimer's disease the nation's third most costly illness, after heart disease and cancer. The Alzheimer's disease research budget has grown substantially over the past decade, to more than $300 million a year. But that figure represents only a small fraction of what the disease costs. The Alzheimer's Association estimates the disease's total cost to American Society at $100 billion a year. I personally think we are at least 10-15 years away from seeing anything really promising.

Leisure time takes on new meaning as does sleep. Messes – remember they are intellectually handicapped. Social life – there is little to none except what you make yourself do. Neighbors – inform them very early on so they can work with you and not against you. You – while you're taking care of the affected individual and managing all the changes that means for your home, family, and finances, you must also carve out time to take care of yourself.

The very week Craig was diagnosed I enrolled him in a drug study. People in the earliest stages of Alzheimer's were much more likely to be treated than those with a more advanced disease. I believe this had no effect on slowing the disease down in Craig but it gave him hope, which was invaluable. I told him he could take two little white pills and he would never be worse than he was that very day. He believed me. Most people with Alzheimer's suffer from depression. Treating their depression also helps preserve their cognitive function. I found it very helpful to make friends with my neighborhood pharmacists and I had a friend who was a medical doctor. Epilepsy drugs may help the agitation as well. Craig did get tremors from time to time and would spill. We tried antidepressants, anti-anxiety drugs and sleeping pills. Each one played a part in helping us to the end.

You need to remember that you are never alone – even when it feels that way. There are people that want to help. You can contact your local Alzheimer's Association, read books – everything. Knowledge is your friend. You cannot be too educated about this disease. The more you know the more you are able to help yourself. We are each our own best friend or our own worst enemy. Make sure that you are your own best friend. Take care of yourself. Caring for someone with Alzheimer's is one of the most challenging roles you will ever have but also one of the most rewarding - knowing that you made a difference. It takes the patience of Job, the Wisdom of Solomon and the selflessness of a saint. Even though few of us have all of these qualities, at some point through the disease you will have been and done each of these. Be a successful caregiver. Take care of yourself. Seek help and don't be afraid to ask. Take time out for yourself – you deserve it. You need and deserve a life of your own. Remember the times when you had little children and you would get a sitter to "take you away" – do it again. Join support groups and listen for advice that others have to share with you. You may be the primary caregiver but you don't have to be the sole caregiver. Don't be a martyr.

Search out care facilities early on so that you are not left with last minute decisions when you are already strained emotionally. It is a tough pill to swallow, but a very necessary one. You could even start early enough to take your loved one with you to observe. I chose not to do this. They don't need to be told what your objectives are. Don't be taken in by colorful literature. Watch and listen to the staff interact with the other residents and how the residents seem to react to them. Talk to the director and to the other staff. Be comfortable with them so they can be comfortable with you. Training is important, but are they kind. Human kindness is so important. You will have everything in writing as you sign contracts for everything you do.

Even into the late stages of Alzheimer's, Craig continued to retain his emotions. He would appear happy, sad, surprised, fearful, worried, angry and depressed. He seemed to recognize people and appear happy most of the time clear up to the last week when his kidneys started to fail and he was in pain. I wanted to be able to donate his brain to science. There was nothing available in the state of Utah that I could find. Universities would take the whole body, but I wasn't ready for that one. I wanted to be able to have closure for me and my family after his death without waiting months for his body to come back. I've found out since that morticians know of other states that will come and harvest the brain and take it to their state. I wished I would have done more homework there. (If this is your desire, talk to your mortician early on to make arrangements) Craig couldn't donate his organs either since we had to wait for him to die and couldn't keep him alive on machines.

Always remember as a caregiver you needn't be alone. Educate yourself, reach out to others and feel the honor in serving this mission you are on. Also, note that November is Alzheimer's month—write letters in your local papers, etc., visit a center and volunteer, seek others out that need help —— but, help. It helps you.

And, now my story about Life with Big Al. . .

August 29, 1996 Craig was diagnosed with Alzheimer's. This is the beginning of our journey along the path known as Alzheimer's…in Craig's case, Early Alzheimer's or as he called it, Big Al. Craig was 52, bright, energetic, independent and very athletic. He had signed a professional baseball contract at 17 years of age. He pursued that dream for seven years. He attended BYU as a business major in the off-season. He spent the rest of that time to the present in retail. The last 11 years he owned his own business.

He worked long hours and ran at least ten miles every day during those last eleven years. He was a marathon runner and an avid golfer. He ran a lot of races from 5K's to marathons. In February of 1993 we went to Las Vegas for a half-marathon. Craig got lost as we were driving back to our hotel. That was unusual for Craig because he had a great sense of direction. That very next week I was diagnosed with Breast Cancer, had a radical mastectomy and went through eight months of Chemotherapy. I spent little to no time at the store with him during this period. I was sick and very weak. The next spring as I was beginning to become myself again, I got an e-coli infection and one of my kidneys failed. I spent weeks in intensive care and it took me a long time to recover again to my whole self. I had always been nicknamed 'double duty Judy'. I tell you these things about myself to help you understand why it took me so long to pick up on things that would have otherwise been obvious to me. I felt that Craig's long hours at the store, long runs and the constant worries about me over the past two years were just taking their toll on him. Little did I realize then that those journeys with Cancer and kidney failure helped prepare me to find the inner strength I would need for this journey with Big Al.

I knew in my heart in April of 1996 that Craig had Alzheimer's. I read and studied everything I could about this disease. I first talked about my fears with a mutual friend, a medical doctor. He agreed to visit Craig while I was in New York and we would talk when I returned. While I was away Craig decided to drive to St. George to golf with some friends. They have since told me that they followed him down and he pulled off the road for reasons they didn't know and then he decided not to play the next day and drove home. When I called from New York and he told me he went to St. George I tried not to react but was frightened as to what could have happened. Craig's driving had made me nervous for quite some time. For at least a three-month period of time I told no one of my fears but was getting calls from friends and also patrons of the store. He would ask people how much change he owed them and then would ask them if the amount he gave them was right. He would tell people that he forgot his glasses (he wore contacts). He covered himself relatively well. I thought about how many people could have taken advantage or perhaps did take advantage of the situation. It got to where I don't know how he operated the cash register, placed the orders, paid invoices or anything else. Craig literally ran the store single-handed with the exception of a few wonderful part-time employees that hold a special place in my heart. One woman said he sold her a pair of shoes for $3 — she must have really thought she was special.

He was losing a contact a week or so he said. He probably just didn't know where he would put them. I would spend approximately 20-30 minutes each night watching him fiddle with them. My heart would be pounding. I'm sure he must have felt as overwhelmed as I did. I would finally tell him that the right lens was in the blue lid and the left in the white lid. I knew that when morning came he wouldn't remember and it didn't matter, because fact of the matter is I didn't know since I couldn't see from my eyes what his eyes needed to see with his lenses. I knew at this point that I needed to help him somehow. I checked into Lasik Surgery. I told them at the clinic of his disease without him knowing. The eye charts were hard. I would have them ask him one row at a time and one letter at a time. I always remained in the room with him. He would get confused when there was too many instructions and too many letters. I was so grateful when the doctor said he was a candidate. We were Federal Expressing a lens in a week at a cost of $106 each. Lasik is considered cosmetic surgery so nothing was covered. (There needs to be circumstances where such things that are necessary for people to function are not considered cosmetic.) This is one of the things we need to work out with insurance as well as having Alzheimer's and other dementia's covered as a disease.

His friends said they wanted to laugh at some of the things he did on the golf course, but at the same time they wanted to cry because they knew something was wrong. He would hit the ball one way, sometimes pick up his clubs, sometimes not, and then walk in the opposite direction. It was almost a relief when we finally had him diagnosed. I say almost...at least we knew what it was and wasn't. I had one doctor talk to him on a referral and Craig told him he thought he had ADD (Attention Deficit Disorder). He had a friend with that and he even gave Craig some of his medicine (Dilantin) to try. It almost made me angry that his friend did. But, I knew he was only trying to help Craig. A lot of his friends were very skeptical. I heard people say they thought I was exaggerating. I don't know why anyone would ever do that. I just wanted people to be aware of this disease and I couldn't by keeping everything to myself. No one could believe Alzheimer's in someone so young and healthy. There were a lot of disbelievers. Because of Craig's activities he had the body and cardiovascular system of a 21-year-old. We sought a medical doctor to eliminate any medical reasons. The doctor asked him the year, who was president, what seven from 100 was, what year he was born and how old he was. I fought back the tears as he answered them wrong. He would practice daily after that for a few weeks. Whatever answer he gave I always told him he was right. He needed constant reassurance that he was okay. I always made sure he got that. Since that time I felt like I buried him a little each day. I feel at times as though I worked three full time jobs and led a double life. I felt like I was in life alone. What I really mean by being in life alone is that I had to make all the day-to-day decisions by myself. Our children were great to help with Craig. Life goes on for everyone as though all of this is not going on around us. Life is for the living. As much as it was nice to have the break away from Craig during the day it was also very hard because it was like leaving your sick child each day. I knew all of the changes that were occurring and what needed to be done for him and with him.

One day he called me after a Chemotherapy treatment to tell me he had lost $6,000. I asked him how he could loose $6,000 and he told me he hadn't lost it he just didn't know where it was. I asked him if he meant in adding/subtracting and he couldn't understand why I would think anything else. I remember going through his books myself even though I was sick. I also should have noticed that his handwriting was getting worse. In April when we had to sign our tax returns, I remember he couldn't get his name on the line where it belonged. He said he couldn't see the small print. It was also in April that I started knowing things weren't right. Each day on his way to the store, he would stop to get a drink and some fruit after his long runs. Several times I would get a call saying he had left the car running and locked the doors and would I come and let him in. I would ask him why he locked the doors with the car running and he would assure me it was because the moneybags were left on the seat.

The girls at the bank would give him a sticker when his deposits were correct. It was almost comical, but sad. I'm sure they had no idea except that he would just get busy and they seemed to be minor mistakes. He put these little stickers on his car window until I took them off. He did tell me that he also had trouble once he got to the drive-up windows knowing what gear to put the car in to pull away. He must have been anxious himself sensing these things going on around him.

I was in ICU (intensive care) with kidney failure and Paul (one of our store employee's) spent the night with me. I'm sure people wondered why Paul spent the night versus Craig. I'm sure he must have wondered the same as myself and we just never communicated it. I think we each thought the same thing at the time. He definitely took charge of the store and Craig. He was a wonder. When anyone would make a comment about Craig and little oddities I would comment that it was all the stress. I thought it was.

We went to Salt Lake to the Expo Mart to market (buying for the store). His driving frightened me and you have to realize that I still had not come to grips with all of this myself let alone talked to our children. I asked if he wanted me to drive. When we arrived we were told that market was the following week. Craig kept questioning the security guard and repeating that his rep wouldn't tell him the wrong week. I didn't know how to let the guard know. I'm sure he wondered about Craig as we walked away. My heart was pounding. We had breakfast at a little sidewalk café and came home – Craig driving.

One of the last times he drove he was following me home from the store and he turned off into the tree streets where he would run. I didn't know at the time I just knew that as I looked in my rearview mirror he was no longer behind me. I waited for what seemed an eternity and he finally arrived home. He got lost, made his way back to the store and then finally home. These were terrifying times because everything was still my little secret that I had not divulged until I knew what I was dealing with. I was also told that he was driving on the wrong side of the road once. I think this frightened him as well and was one of the reasons he gave up driving so willingly. He would still ask to drive once in a while. I would take him to the empty parking lot where our store was located and let him drive around. One Sunday he started going a little fast as I watched him and I thought to myself, who am I kidding. He is sick and I should not allow him behind the wheel.

I read and studied everything I could. I found out that early Alzheimer patients usually go faster and that the life expectancy is 3-10 years with exceptions along the way. After the medical doctor we had to go to a neurologist and have an MRI to eliminate the diagnosis of a brain tumor. I asked for an extra copy of the MRI and studied it myself at home. I had studied pictures of healthy brains versus dementia type diseased brains. You could see the atrophy on both sides of his brain. We had a clinical psychologist (August 29, 1996) do the testing and it was a horrendous nightmare for Craig — very humiliating for him and heartbreaking for me. It was hard for him to realize he no longer knew his address or phone or what year it was. It took him over two hours instead of one because Craig would keep telling him he wasn't quite ready. It was a Mini-Mental State Examination. Craig's remote memory was still pretty good. He would tell people that he never was good in school and all he did was play baseball. In reality Craig was a very good student even throughout his college years. In fact as I think back when he thought he was depressed or anxious I wonder if he was experiencing symptoms then but didn't know how to identify what was happening to him. His vocabulary was the only function that had been spared. His dramatic loss in intellectual ability is seen in 'advanced' stages of dementia of the Alzheimer's type. The clinical psychologist then asked Craig to wait out front while he talked to me. He told me to read the book *The 36-Hour*

Day: A Family Guide to Caring for Persons with Alzheimer Disease, Related Dementing Illnesses, and Memory Loss in Later Life by Nancy L. Mace, Peter V. Rabins and Paul R. McHugh, published by Johns Hopkins University Press, which I had already read. I knew what was ahead. I was grateful that I had been resourceful to have read and understood about his diagnosis and was as prepared as I could have been. I gained my composure, wiped away my tears and we went out to the waiting room. Craig was not there. He had run home through the park. My heart raced and I said a million prayers to not cry. I went through the door and Craig was standing there crying. We held each other for what seemed an eternity. Oh, what heartache. He said please don't ever do that to me again. I promised I wouldn't. Craig went through a period of depression after that. It was at that point that I knew I needed to do something — but what? I learned of a study group in drug research. Because Craig was relatively young, 52, and healthy, he was a prime candidate for a study. We were accepted, Craig as the patient and me as the "competent caregiver." I told him that we were very lucky because of the fact that he was young and healthy that he would never be any worse than he was that day and that if we could make it through my Cancer we could make it through this. And, that if this is as bad as it got we could handle that and it was my turn to take care of him like he took care of me. We held each other and cried. To me this seemed the kind thing to do because as he declined he wouldn't know it. This was my "Craig Graduation" plan. This was the plan that seemed to evoke care and understanding for the person I loved the most. I use the word "graduation" knowing that Alzheimer's is fatal with no cures, no hope, no anything. So, I wanted to make the most of the time we had together until he "graduated" from this earth and this life and moved on to the next and I would be responsible for filling that time. I know that my life was spared for some reason and this must be it. I knew I would be able to do it and be blessed. I know some material you read says to involve the person so you can make decisions about their care early on. I couldn't imagine letting him know that he would require resthome care and probably not know us. He would tell people he took two little white pills and he'd be the same forever. I had an attorney draw up new wills including a living will for each of us. I knew Craig would not want to be kept alive by machines. It was at this point that papers were drawn up also that I would be Craig's legal guardian and had Power of Attorney. This was hard for me to do. In fact, I went to the attorney's office and he asked where Craig was. I told him I left him home and would just take the papers for him to sign. I was so nervous. I almost felt dishonest knowing what I was doing without saying anything about what he was signing. He reminded me that his signature or what there was left of his signature needed to be notarized. He gave me a hug and I went back and got Craig. There was a terrible snowstorm and I remember sliding all over the road on my way home to get him. When I got back I told Craig I had forgotten that I had made an appointment with Doug, his friend, to have new wills made up for the two of us. I felt better having that behind me. I was now Craig's legal guardian. I no longer needed to worry that he was unable to sign his name. I could/would sign it for him and it was my signature that was now his legal signature. People never ceased to be amazed that found out. Craig has always been the epitome of health and fitness — both mentally and physically. I felt the way I handled it was the humane/kind way to approach Big Al.

One of the neurologists I saw told me that he would be surprised if Craig lasted three years and it would be a blessing if he didn't. I cried a lot. Alzheimer's is an ugly disease. As I read and studied I believe that not only are you robbed of your loved one, but also they rob you of whatever you have worked your whole life for and from this point forward you've lost their income as well. No care is covered with Alzheimer's. It is from this time forward that you continually lose a little more of them each day.

Our children handled it relatively well. I had to remind myself that I had been preparing and studying for months about Alzheimer's and had time to let it sink in. I had a knot in my stomach and cried a lot when I was alone. So, I knew the children would have to go through this same grieving period. It's like I said earlier, you bury them a little every day. I think more so in the beginning and then you let it go until the latter part of the disease. It's looking at it as being able to say a long good-bye and it's hard. The children and I grieved and cried a lot in the beginning. I remember picking my daughter, Suzanne, and her children up and going to one of Steve's (my son) job sites to tell him. He had a staple gun and he took the children and let them shoot it into the ground as we all cried. It was very hard for all of us that day as we all contemplated what was ahead of us or more importantly what was ahead for Craig. Craig spent probably the first three to four weeks at home and not going to the store much during the initial "start" period. We decided that as a family we would laugh instead of cry and keep him home for as long as we could possibly care for him ourselves. Craig would constantly joke about "Big Al."

He would need the light on at night because he would get so turned around. He didn't know where his head went versus his feet in bed. I tried to make things as easy as possible by being in bed first and having the covers turned down. For some reason his feet would itch and he would like me to spray them with a foot spray before going to bed. We developed new little rituals. He could no longer stand to urinate so I would remind him to pull his pants down and just sit. The only difference between Craig and a little child is that Craig didn't know where the toilet was even when you pointed to it. You would have to turn him around and help him sit down. Going to bed was pretty much the same way. He didn't know how to lay his head down, where it was supposed to go and then cover up.

We are into the **end of May, 1997** and he was becoming more confused about days and he described that next day by "after we sleep again then it will be ___." One morning as we awoke he looked at me and said, "Now I forget, how are we related?" I knew this would come but it still shocked me. I turned away for a minute to gather my thoughts and asked him back, "How do you think we are related?" He didn't know and I told him we were married. I was afraid of more questions, got out of bed to fix breakfast and turned the television on for him.

Our son, Steve, wanted to spend a week golfing with him back in the Carolinas where he used to be a golf professional. So, Steve and his family, Wendy, Taylor, Madison, Craig and myself went back to South Carolina and spent a week with friends. We all had a wonderful time; especially Craig. I'm so glad Steve insisted that we go. When I look back and discover that all we have in the end is our memories I feel very fortunate. Just like the perfect sunset never quite leaves our consciousness our memories are the same, always there to draw upon.

When he wanted me to read the scriptures to him we read for a few days. He decided he didn't like that book very well and asked if we could find another one. We graduated to Gospel Doctrine and lasted for a few more days. It was at this point that I got the animated version of the

Bible and Book of Mormon on videotape. There was a pioneer documentary with them as well but unanimated. That was his favorite and he wished the others were like that one. He watched that one a lot.

Sundays seemed to be his favorite day and I thought it was because of church, but I discovered it was because I never left him on Sundays and I was his security blanket.

The store was getting harder for him and harder for the employees. It was like leading a double life. I told him what he needed to hear and then do whatever I needed him to do for the sake of the store. It is stressful because I almost think that he knows what's going on. He appears to be so normal at times. I let him talk me into ordering a bunch of a certain brand of shoes. I should have known better and he would never have known. We would tell him we did whatever he asked us to and then make up some excuse as to why after. We had to keep reminding ourselves that because he looked like he was fine – he wasn't and the only real working part of his brain was his verbal skills. I would have to keep reminding myself of the tests and the wrong answers to them.

Suzanne and her family moved into a home in our neighborhood. This was a godsend in our life for her to be close and help me care for her father even though we told him it was because he needed to help her with Alex and Emily since she was pregnant. He thought it was great that he could help. And, since his children were everything in the world to him he was only too happy to help. He told me it was hard being a helper all the time and babysitting. One day he said it was my turn to play Barbie's with Emily, who was three.

I offered our son in-law, Stephen, a salary if he would start January 1st and manage the store. I couldn't handle not knowing if I had an employee to show up at 10:00 while I needed to be to work everyday myself. We needed my paycheck and I needed my health insurance. I could finally leave for work every morning and know that everything would be taken care of. All of the reps from the various companies have been great to work with me and now our son in-law in Craig's absence. What was hard was that Craig could talk with someone for a short period of time and you would think that everything was okay. It is just being around him for periods of time that you would soon realize it was not.

He usually put his underclothes on backwards. I would tell him it was because I forgot to turn them right side out when I put them away or I put them backward in the drawer. We had two sizes of clothes. On the day he thought he was a little heavy we would go for the 34 otherwise we did the 33. I eventually got 36's. He loved three-quarter arch supports for his shoes and couldn't have enough. I kept a pair in a box because he always wanted a new pair and I would just rotate the ones we had. He always thought his shoes were 'flat' without them.

On most nights he didn't want to take a whole sleeping pill so I told him I "slivered" it. We both needed our sleep. One night I gave him one in some raspberry tea I made. I've decided you need to do whatever it takes each day to make it through to the next. Suzanne came over one night when we were having tea and she asked me if we were 'dosing' and Craig wondered what that meant and I explained it was just the kind of tea we were drinking.

Steve took his dad with him from time to time and told him he was going to get a leash for him so he wouldn't lose him and then they both laughed. Craig was aware that he got turned around, he just didn't know the extent of it. It was frightening. I didn't dare leave his side in a store. He would be gone in a flash and you wouldn't know where he was. And, it was impossible to yell his name when you've got this grown-up person that looked perfectly normal.

July 20, 1997. *"Let not your heart be troubled: ye believe in God, believe also in me. In my Father's house are many mansions: if it were not so, I would have told you. I go to prepare a place for you. And if I go and prepare a place for you I will come again, and receive you unto myself; that where I am, there ye may be also."* (John 14:1-3) — We went to a restaurant with the children for Steve's birthday. Craig had trouble with buffets. They are becoming more and more confusing to him. He rode to Salt Lake with the girls and myself (I needed shoes and he couldn't figure out why). He is nervous in crowds. He is moving slower. Escalators (he called them alligators) make him very uneasy. I think the only reason he went with us is that I was the security blanket. He feels safe and secure when I'm around. He's become more unsure of his footing. He is not real coherent in his thought pattern and words are sometimes harder to come by. I try not to fill in the blanks too soon for him.

July 21, 1997. *"Today is the first day of the rest of my life"* — His friend, Jesse took him to lunch today. They went to a diner. He said he sent the food back three times because it wasn't hot enough. He says that a lot about the food being cold or not hot enough. We had waffles with the children tonight. He didn't want any. He doesn't like sweet things anymore. He had a bad headache all day and noise seems to bother him a lot. I called him to tell him I was bringing lunch and he said he was talking to the prophet (he was watching the church president on television). He gets confused with words. He tells people that he can't eat sugar anymore since the disease. We just tell him that whatever it is that he wants to eat has no sugar and then he eats it. Suzanne took him to a movie this afternoon, *GI Jane*. She's brave because not only is a theatre dark but there are stairs involved that he can't navigate. She said he would talk out loud and keep asking if people knew if that was a guy or was it really a girl. We both laughed and cried when they returned home.

August 1, 1997. *"I will be as kind and forgiving as I want others to be toward me"* — One of the things I've learned is to not say anything until right before the time to go or do. He seems to have no concept of time anymore. It's good to have made arrangements in advance without his knowledge of someone to pick him up for lunch or golf. He can still golf, but it's getting harder. He thinks he could do better if I would just organize his clubs and find someone to give him lessons. Craig was a championship golfer. He talks about his disease freely to folks and he calls it "Big Al". Suzanne said he was washing his golf balls off in the toilet. She asked what he was doing and he said that he was getting his balls cleaned in the sink. Bill picked him up to play golf (hit balls). He was trying to help Craig and told him you needed to keep everything 'square' - and square it was. Everything to Craig from that day on was 'square' – it didn't matter what you were talking about. I would never have figured it out. Bill and Doris took us to dinner one Sunday and he started talking about 'square' and I just shrugged my shoulders like I didn't know what he was talking about. And, then Bill told me the story of how he lined him up with the golf club and his shoulders and he was 'square'....

He continued to run each day. Craig would run up to ten miles per day. One day he ran for four hours, but he said he wasn't lost. The children and I think he was but didn't know so he kept on running until he found a location familiar and found his way home. I enrolled him in the "Lost Program" – for Alzheimer's. He wore a necklace that identified him as memory impaired. Craig could not read from the earliest diagnosis of his disease. So, I told him that his necklace told people that he took medicine and it was very important to always wear it.

One day Craig went to eat with friends after golfing. He came home and told me what he did and I asked him what he ate. He said he couldn't remember but he had one of those drinks that his friend has. I quizzed him a little to see what it was and we decided it was coffee. He looked a little befuddled and said, "oh, I shouldn't have liked that because I think I'm not supposed to drink that". We both chuckled and I said I didn't think it mattered much. I assured him everything was fine and it was hot chocolate. He said, "wow, that's a relief."

A co-worker went with me to visit two care centers. It was a hard day. One was like a total resthome atmosphere and the other one was a daycare center for only ten Alzheimer patients. These were hard times as I was doing things so foreign. Things you had never even imagined doing for a parent let alone a spouse and a healthy 53-year-old. I took Craig for a half day to the daycare center for Alzheimer patients and he wasn't pleased. When I picked him up he told me they were all "older than dirt" and asked me if I knew that? I acted like I didn't and asked him what they ate for lunch. He told me "worms" — I said you mean spaghetti and he said no it was yellow and that I should know because I am the one that likes it. I said Fettuccini and that wasn't right either. We finally decided that it was macaroni and cheese and he said the lady that made it said it wasn't good either that it wasn't just him. Needless to say we have not been back yet.

August 15, 1997. *"Birth is the gateway to mortal life – death is the gateway to immortality and eternal life"* — I even got up the courage to visit the cemetery. I'm proud of myself to think I have been doing things I would never have to do until I was old(er). I drove to the cemetery three times before I got the courage to go in and talk to the Sexton. Even after they showed me the available plots it took me another two weeks to go look at them and make the purchase. The plots depended on whether we would have flat headstones or upright. I bought two plots that could have either one we wanted because I didn't want to pick out the headstone yet. I hope to do that one of these days soon. I would like the children to help me with this one so it will have to wait.

Suzanne tends her Dad every day. She has been a wonder. Having her husband, Stephen, work at the store and still be able to take Craig once in a while works out very well. We have told him that while she is pregnant she needs help with her two little ones so that he will not want to go to the store. They spent the summer going to the zoo, parks, picnics and lots of fun things. Craig still thinks that he was the helper. On the day at the zoo she had him push Emily and she pushed Alex. He was so intent on watching her and not getting lost that he forgot Emily and left her at the polar bears. A gentleman asked him if he didn't forget something. Craig just looked puzzled. Suzanne had him go back and get Emily and had her eyes on both of them. One of the things with this disease is that people around don't understand when a grown person who looks young and healthy does strange things. Another day they went to an art museum and Suzanne told her dad they were ready to go and he was staring at a painting on the wall and talking to the guy in the painting (George Washington crossing the Delaware). He talked to him like he was living and said, "boy, buddy I bet you're cold."

It is harder for him to use a public restroom. He gets confused with the doors and even more confused when he sees himself in the mirror. He thinks someone is in there with him.

A neighbor runs with him each morning. It has gotten to where Craig, who used to run at least 10 miles a day, is outrun by someone who is just a casual runner. He has been great to help. It's nice to have someone you know you can depend on that isn't frightened by the situation. His own father passed away with Alzheimer's. Craig feels comfortable with their family. He is used to seeing them each day because they do our yardwork.

November 10, 1997. *"Hardships and trials are gifts"*— I am determined to write daily about Craig to keep a record for our grandchildren about a grandfather that loved them so very much. Craig's children and grandchildren are the most important assets he has. They are his crowning jewels. Craig seems to be slipping rapidly. He gets confused about eating. He doesn't know if he just ate or needs to eat. He sometimes thinks that once he has a bowel movement he no longer has any food in his system and he needs to eat again. He gets agitated easily and moves slowly when he walks. He seems to talk louder too. He doesn't know enough to slide his chair to the table when we eat. You have to slide the table to him and then he still spills on himself. I try to make our dinner time quiet and simple. When there are too many plates on the table he gets confused as to which one he should eat off of. I make sure we each have one plate and there is nothing else on the table – simplicity.

He continually asks me how we are related and how old we are. Tonight he needed to urinate and had me go with him because he said he didn't remember what to do. I finally had him sit on the toilet and thought it would be better because he seems to get wet and it frustrates him. I give him Seconol (a sleeper) about 8:00 and then by 9:00 he is ready to go to bed. If I'm tired I'll stay in bed and if not or I've got a lot to do I get back up after I know he is sound asleep. This helps me keep sane in this new world of repetitiveness and continual questions. Our children are fantastic to help and I could not have made it through this last year without them, but I also believe they have a life with their mates and children and they can help, but I need to make most of the choices and do most of the caring myself. I feel like I have enough common sense I will know when the time is right that Craig will need more help than I can give him.

November 11, 1997. *"All that we have left when we leave this earth is how much we have loved others"* — Craig spent the morning with his sister. She then took him up to his mother's. Suzanne picked him up and brought him home. He is becoming more repetitive and asking more questions all the time. He's having more of a struggle with going to the bathroom without help.

November 12, 1997. *"Joy is found in the love we give and friendships we make"* — Craig spent the morning with his mother and then Steve picked him up for lunch. I got a call at work saying there was an emergency. Craig was literally falling apart — crying and saying he wanted to kill himself. Steve and I ate lunch and discussed possible plans to take as we go forward. Steve is worried that I'm going to break down. I almost believe Craig heard us.

November 13, 1997. *"Our fortunes are in how we think and feel"* — He keeps crying and asks if I am going to put him away somewhere? He's cried all day again. I gave him a triple dose of Ativan (an anti-anxiety medication) today and last night I called the pharmacist and asked if he could take a double dose of his sleeping medication. Yes. Now it makes me a little nervous for tomorrow morning. I don't know how long I can continue to be tough or strong. I am waiting for the neurologist, to call me back to discuss options I have with Craig for medication, anti-depressants, whatever??? He never did call back. It was at this point I decided you need to read, study and become friends with your neighborhood pharmacist. You are the one to determine your loved one's needs. When I say their needs you need to consider your needs. You need to consider what they need to help you get through this as well. We need to educate ourselves as much as possible with every aspect of the disease and medications that will help.

I had Suzanne watch her Dad for a half-hour while I ran to the store and when I got back he had come back to our house to use the bathroom. I don't know what went wrong but his shirt and pants were in the hall along with his shoes and socks. His underclothes were all wet and the water in the tub was running and he had a bowel movement. I don't know if he had it in his shorts and was trying to clean it up or what and I guess I will never know, but it was everywhere. I just threw everything out and washed him off and put clean clothes on. I talked about pleasant things, got us some food to eat and we talked a little more and then at 7:00 he said he wanted to go to bed. Craig never goes to bed alone anymore. Just another thing that he is not himself. I suppose this is more of the disease as it takes over his mind. I hope and pray to stay strong.

November 16, 1997. *"Birth and death are the starts of new journeys"* — Craig started on anti-depressants yesterday. I've decided that since I did not get a response from the neurologist I would go directly to my doctor friend. He is the one that I first confided in or talked to when I reached the conclusion of Alzheimer's. We decided that between the two of us we could do what we needed to help Craig reach graduation day and keep myself sane and together in the process. I've decided that it will be a bittersweet day. I feel that I lost Craig a long time ago. I also feel that

Craig and I have had a better 34 years together than those who have been able to celebrate their Golden wedding anniversary together. Craig and I have gotten along so well through the years. I only remember two real arguments and the one I remember him laughing at me and it made me feel terrible and I cried. He said he had never seen me angry and laughed more. We communicated well. We were just two people that did not argue. Steve and Suzanne could not have had a more loving father that taught them love, patience, and kindness. Craig also taught them the honor of hard work and honesty with others and more importantly, yourself.

November 17, 1997. *"I will set aside my unhappy feelings and begin anew to face the problems of the day"* — Craig spent the day with Suzanne and her children. They went to visit his mother in the afternoon. It was Madison's third birthday on Saturday and we waited until tonight to take our gift. We had such a fun time. It thrills us both to see Steve with his two children. He is such a good dad. Craig gets teary eyed every time we leave their home. He is always praising Steve and always saying he couldn't have done it without Wendy. He dearly loves them. Craig loves being a father and grandfather.

Our neighbors, the Stringhams, came down tonight and watched him for an hour. I went to pick up his prescription of Paxil (20 mg) and Seconal (100 mg). Paxil is an anti-depressant and we are trying that twice a day in place of the Ativan (1/2 mg). I give him the Seconal (a sleeper) around 7:30-8:30. On some nights I give him two. I've decided it doesn't matter what he gets addicted to...whatever helps us reach past to the next day in as little as anxiety as possible.

When I think back about the trips that we took with the company I work for and he had a hard time pronouncing Nanaimo. We all laughed, but it was more than that. We sold our Ford Bronco II to a friend and then Craig wanted to finance getting it back. I thought he was crazy, but just was attached to the car, and he bought it back only to sell it again. When we went to the Boulders in Arizona he and another spouse went to a store while we had a meeting, he drove and was on the wrong side of the road. He told her he just couldn't see at night. I think she was aware there was something wrong too. A friend called me at work to tell me that patrons of the store were calling him with concerns and he didn't know how to approach me but straight on. Oh, these little things that should have been so obvious.

November 19, 1997. *"A father's legacy is measured by the deeds of his children"* — I don't know how I have managed to stay sane and survive these past few years. Between the anxiety at work and everything about the store we own and life in general, it's overwhelming if I allow it to be. Our children have been 'godsends' in my life.

I feel scattered on some days but not depressed. I get physically exhausted at times. It is hard to get Craig up and literally place him in front of his food and make sure he's eating. I have been using an electric razor to shave him and decided I didn't like it very well. So, one morning I called Steve and asked if I went up or down, and then went for the real razor. I did a great job and Craig looked and I think even felt better. I have to place everything in front of him, including turning the water on. I then tell him to take his clothes off, turn the shower on and help him in. I have to tell him to pick the soap up and I shampoo his hair. He can partially dry himself and I finish up. He can no longer figure out how to clothe himself. Sometimes he can put on his own socks and shoes and sometimes not. Tonight he couldn't even take his own shoes and socks off and he was extremely anxious.

November 20, 1997. *"A true friend is an angel in disguise"* — I took the day off. I went to work for two hours and had Craig stay with Suzanne. I came home for an hour and we had lunch together with Suzanne and our little grandson. We then ran a few errands together and Craig actually came with me to get my hair cut. The girl that cuts my hair washes Craig's hair and trims it up every Wednesday. She has been so sweet. Craig loves it that she pampers him. One morning when he was sitting on the bed and I was brushing his hair for him he noticed himself in the mirror. He said he looked like a stud since she had been doing his hair and getting rid of all that fluff in the back. He then said that probably wasn't nice to say (calling himself a stud). Craig has always been shy and quiet. Never one to call attention to himself. He has always been immaculate with himself. I try to have him look every day like he would if it were years back and he was doing this for himself. I know that he would do the same for me.

He is always thanking me and is so appreciative for all the little things I do. I've noticed that he is constantly telling me how much he loves me and doesn't know what he would do without me.

One night we were sitting in front of the television and he wanted to know what I had done with all of his running medals (he's won a lot of road races). He said that when he dies he wants his grandchildren to have those. Every once in a while he comes out with a strange comment like that. He asked about his old baseball bats that have his signature on them because he wanted each of his children to have one. He can carry on a conversation relatively well at times and then not be able to walk up a flight of stairs by himself. It is, indeed, a strange disease.

November 21, 1997. *"If you want to leave your footprints, wear your workshoes"* — He said he didn't feel well when I wanted him to stay with his mother. It was almost like he was having an anxiety attack. Camille washed and cut his hair again. He loves it. He called her a 'babe' as she told him how nice it was that he let her cut his hair. I think the comment shocked us both and we chuckled. She said none of her clients had ever called her that before. He spent the morning with his sister and all the way to her house told me thanks for letting him go with me yesterday to get his hair cut and how fun it was to watch me and that I just got cuter every day. I told him that people don't get cuter as they get older, but he said I did. I laughed all the way to his sister's house and I almost think I was embarrassed.

November 22, 1997. *"Life is a grindstone, whether it grinds you down or polishes you up, depends on what you are made of"* — He went to the BYU/Utah game today with friends. He stayed the whole game and did great. They had taken him twice and I know that it isn't easy because it is like baby-sitting. I'm so appreciative of his friends that are willing to take him places and help him. It certainly makes my day easier. I call each of them my "missionary companions" on this journey. With all my heart I want to do this well and walk hand in hand with Craig until we reach graduation day. He deserves the very best. I want to understand this disease all that I can.

November 23, 1997. *"The depth of our gratitude is the depth of our understanding"* — Wendy and the girls stopped by this morning to visit. Madison wanted to stay and go to church with us. So they all stayed and went to church. We had to go 20 minutes early — because if you don't you can't get a parking place close and it's too hard to have Craig walk very far. Craig got a little anxious on the way home. Occasionally, he says he feels funny and I never quite know what that means.

November 25, 1997. *"You can eat an elephant if you just eat him a bite at a time"* — Craig spent the day with Suzanne. He enjoys his time with her. Jesse picked him up and took him to lunch. He said he even helped him eat. He just needs help making sure that he holds the sandwich right so it doesn't fall everywhere. He likes to keep money in his pockets. He doesn't know what he does with it so I only put a few ones unless he needs more to go with someone for lunch and he likes to feel he is paying his way. He also has hemorrhoids again. We go through a lot of hemorrhoid cream. Whenever someone takes him to lunch he is so appreciative that he wants me to call him or her and tell them thanks or he wants me to send a thank you card.

November 26, 1997. *"Strength comes from your heart"* — Wednesday before Thanksgiving — Craig called it Turkey Day. I went to work for only a few hours this morning and Craig stayed with Suzanne and the children. I went to the shoe store and talked with the employees. I let them know the extent of Craig's deterioration and each one of them wanted to help. I'm so appreciative of these young people and their goodness. Pat, Vaughn and Paige all worked with Craig when he was well. They are each my companions. I returned home and stayed with Craig and the children while Suzanne ran an errand for me. I decided to get three little log pole trees in place of a Christmas tree and then just put little white lights on them. Craig has hemorrhoids again pretty bad and doesn't quite understand what to do. He can no longer sit down into the tub and get out on his own so I just had him stand in a hot shower tonight for as long as he could. He is also having little accidents more often. I'm glad that we have these next few days home together in the mornings and not have to rush anywhere. I am so appreciative this Thanksgiving for the wonderful blessings that God has given me, Craig being at the top of the list.

November 28, 1997. *"Let your light so shine before men, that they may see your good works, and glorify your Father which is in Heaven" (Matthew 5:16)* — Friday night - the night after Thanksgiving. We spent the day with family and friends. I got Craig in a hot tub tonight (I called our neighbor first to see if her husband was there if I needed help getting him out). Then I went for it knowing that he would help. He keeps telling me he is an athlete and can do anything. It took three attempts and two near misses at falling back but we made it. I thought there for a minute that he would fall back and crack his head – which would be all we would need. He doesn't understand how to get up after he is sitting down and he's too heavy for me to lift and the tub being slippery frightens him. He wants me to get a new "bottom" in the tub that works better than the one we have.

November 29, 1997. *"I am dedicated to learning something new each day"* — If Craig could go back in time I'm sure he wouldn't change too many things. His life was and is the monument he left. His path has always been on the straight and narrow. Towards the end of his earthly life the path got a little rough — a little bumpy — perhaps rockier for us as we watched him stumble along the rocks and gravel that were strewn along the home stretch. Your heart aches so much inside that you want to protect him. He twitches a lot. This morning I almost got a speeding ticket. It took me so long to get him ready and then myself and I was running late. I got pulled over and jumped out of the car close to tears and knew that Craig could not see me cry nor let the officer say where my thoughts were with Craig and Alzheimer's. The officer told me to get back into the car and I explained quickly why I got out first. I then got back into the car and the officer knew Craig and told him he just stopped us to say 'hello' and see how he was doing. I was so relieved and appreciative. Craig thought that was so nice of him to recognize us and do that. Tonight I made him toast (he likes that at night lately) and some hot chocolate. I only fill his cup half full now in case he twitches it doesn't spill as bad. I almost gave him grape juice tonight and decided against it.

Smart move — he spilled the hot chocolate on the couch, his legs and slippers. He doesn't know how to pronounce toast (dose) but I've gotten better at interpreting.

The anti-depressants are working pretty well. He doesn't seem to get so anxious and doesn't see "snow" or hallucinate as much. He still says he feels water drops on his arms and hands at times. The pills must make his mouth dry and he likes to chew gum, but he doesn't know to throw it away or where to spit it out, and the last time it went on the rug. So, I'm careful that I'm around when he gets gum. It's always the little things that you know and don't tell everyone that you feel protective about. I took him to the grocery store and he was behind me in the line and pointing to the gum asking if he could have some. The checker knew he had Alzheimer's and told him she was sure Judy would let him have whatever kind he wanted. He looked at me to get approval and picked up two packs.

November 30, 1997. *"Nurture your family garden with tender loving care"* — Craig became nervous and anxious again this morning. I talked him into going to the first part of church. The neighbor boys take turns staying home with him. They have been great. We all went to dinner tonight after church. We had a nice visit and a few laughs. Craig asked our neighbor if he would take him to go "tinkle" — the boys just chuckled. (For two young boys I have been impressed with their kindness and understanding towards Craig.) I ran to grab them to let our neighbor know about having him sit versus standing to urinate and Craig was already starting to undo his pants before they got through the door. He can't use public restrooms by himself anymore. One thing I have learned is that people don't have a clue about what is going on. For the most part people don't realize the extent of Craig's decline because he looks healthy and I always have him dressed nice, shaved and groomed well.

Craig spent the morning with his mother and she helped him again with hot compresses for his hemorrhoids. He wanted to call her all night to thank her. He is very appreciative of everything that everyone does for him. He constantly says thanks and tells me he loves me. He gets nervous or anxious if I am not in bed with him when he wakes up. Some nights when I move to the other bedroom to get some sleep as soon as I hear him move around I hurry back to our bed so he'll go back to sleep. It is much like a little child. You need to be there by their side to reassure them you are there and everything is all right.

December 4, 1997. *"True friends are never acquired by chance, they are always gifts from God"* — I gave Craig two sleeping pills last night so when he woke up and ate breakfast he wanted to lay back down and sleep. I took a half-day of vacation and stayed home with him this morning. His friends, Bob and Richard, picked him up and took him to lunch. He was nervous to go because he is afraid to use a public restroom. Jesse called and wanted to take him to lunch as well and he talked on the phone with him for a while. They are very kind to Craig. His friend, Mel, called to check on him tonight and offered to take him to lunch tomorrow. Craig is becoming more disoriented and able to do fewer things for himself. I watch him eat and he hardly knows how to pick a sandwich up and eat it anymore. I've tried flat flour tortillas filled and rolled. I would put a napkin around it to hold the bottom but he would start to eat the paper before I could undo it. He still remembers most people, things and places. Sometimes I think his memory is better than mine. Work is a little crazy. I feel a little overwhelmed. My mind feels like it is running overtime. I want to sit and cry, but know that I need to be tough and stay together for the two of us. Craig talks a lot about going to St. George next year to play golf and about getting his act together to run more every day. The reality of it is that I am afraid to let him go run by himself anymore. It is so cold outside that if he got lost it would frighten me. He is going to run Saturday morning with the race team and our neighbor (we co-sponsor a running race team with a major shoe manufacturer). As hard as it is to get him into a tub it seems to relax him at night so I have continued to do that. I wish I could get a video of him trying to sit down and then trying to get out. It's hard to imagine that the mind can forget a simple thing as sitting and then getting back up. I often wonder what would happen or where he would be at today if he knew the reality of this disease and where he is really going to be at next year. It truly is a reality that there are new beginnings at the end of life. As we face death we learn more about life and living and the important things of loving each other daily. We can't relive our lives but it's wonderful that we can learn from our experiences. It is said that life must be understood backwards. But we forget the other proposition, that it must be lived forwards. What a world this would be if we did know in the beginning what we know in the end. Our suffering can be turned into a celebration of the sweetness of human life.

Craig, out of the blue, will ask me questions or talk about someone and I won't have a clue what or who he is talking about. I always act like I do and a lot of times it is like Charades. Some of our friends are pretty good at the game with him.

I've decided to keep the shoe store for the time being and have our son in-law continue to manage it and send letters out to friends, schools, peace officers, etc. that need athletic shoes and let them know our intentions to help them and hope that they continue to help us be a successful independent business. Craig has worked hard over the last ten years to make the store succeed. As one of our race team members said he is something like an icon and his name is connected with the store.

I wish that I could go to bed at night and forget everything and turn my mind off and awake the next morning to face a new day, which is unlike the one we left behind. Each day is a new learning with Craig as to where he/we will be at on that day. They say that each day for the Alzheimer patient is a new day unlike any other. It is also the same for the Caregiver.

December 7, 1997. *"If tragedy drops you to your knees, then it becomes a victory"* — We had a long day - too long. Craig was crying, needing to eat again and more. It seems as when he gets sick or frightened he thinks he needs to eat. I don't know what is going on in his brain, but he thinks food is going to make him feel better. I've decided no physical illness could be worse than when your mind goes. On some days it is so hard to keep up the facade that he is healthy and we are going to grow old together and retire. We went to three hours of church, went to eat with Bill and Doris and then went to see the Christmas lights in Mapleton and in Spanish Fork. It was too much and too long of a day for Craig and I should have known better. He cried for Suzanne and said I was mad at him because he needed more food. I try to talk him out of eating so much because it's so hard for him to eat and then he thinks I don't believe him that he is sick — oh, if he only knew. Some days it is so trying that I just don't know what to do. Some days I feel as if I'm Super Woman and other days I wonder how and what am I doing. Tonight when we changed his clothes and put his robe and slippers on he wanted new underclothes on and he tried to put his bottoms on his head. We both laughed. He tells me his slippers are just getting too flat. With his shoes he has arch supports and he gets confused with his slippers because they are "flat". I told him that Santa could bring us new slippers for Christmas. He actually spilled hot chocolate on his slippers one night, so he needs new ones. Although he has no idea of Christmas or what it means.

I've decided that the less confusion and the more simple the day, the better Craig is. I noticed that even sitting on the second row in our Sunday school class he felt too enclosed or claustrophobic. I've decided we need to sit on the front ends and then it's not like we've got so many people around us.

I sometimes wish that Craig did not have such a healthy body. He is always so thoughtful and kind, generous and caring. He's always very appreciative of everything you do for him, but every now and then I get a glimpse of someone that gets upset with me when he thinks he's feeling sick and not knowing what is going on and he's telling me he needs to eat more. I've actually given him two sleeping tablets tonight so I don't know what tomorrow morning will bring, but I also know that I do what I need to do at the time. I've decided that if this is my mission on this earth that I have to take one day at a time and that the Lord is going to provide a way for me to make it to the next and everything will work out for the best.

December 8, 1997. *"Bloom where you are planted"* — Today I took a day of vacation and stayed home with Craig. He slept most of the day away. With two sleeping pills and up and down all night I just let him sleep. Today was hard. Steve called this morning to check on things and said that somedays it just doesn't seem fair – Dad is the most kind and loving person I know. I try so hard every day to look at this as a mission and a blessing that we will all learn from and be better people because of having Craig touch our life and being able to help him to graduate from this earthly life. I only wish graduation day and those wings could come sooner for him rather than later. I don't even feel guilty when I think it or say it anymore because in some ways I think Craig is so aware at times and it is hard on him as well. He asks me a lot about the disease and why he can't get out of the tub as fast as me or why he gets so anxious. I always reassure him.

He seems to get headaches a lot lately. I don't know if it is the anti-depressants, sleeping medication or what. I remembered a thought once about death and sleep. It is said that you sleep a lot at the end as you prepare for your final rest. I hope to be brave and able to endure and not become overwhelmed with everything. I think if we were older, closer to retirement, I could stay home with him. If we were debt free and knew we had an income monthly that the days would be easier to swallow. As I think about my Breast Cancer, I think how strong I was, and now as I look back it was nothing compared to what we face with this. At least there is a treatment or cure to try for Cancer. I hope that by donating Craig's brain to science that it will help determine clues for someone else. There needs to be a way to keep them alive to harvest their organs when they are young and healthy. What a wonderful thought that lives could be saved or prolonged. Craig has so enriched my life and others and how wonderful it would be if he could have passed the gift of life on to others. I know as I write this that some might think it morbid, but I have had at least two years now to think about this and I feel as I bury Craig a little each day as I lose him a little each day. I will always have my Craig in the eternities and in my memories.

December 11, 1997. *"The city of happiness is found in the state of the mind"* — Craig has decided to ride the "horse" stationary bike every morning and night. After 10-20 minutes he tells people he rides for an hour and a half. This morning he told me we had to talk. He proceeded to tell me we had not had sex in ten years and wondered if I had a boyfriend. I told him he was my only boyfriend. He got a funny look on his face and said, "oh, my gosh, you like girls." I assured him I did not like anyone except him. I tried to assure him it hasn't been that long. He says he has a good memory and he even writes it down. This is a period of our life that is gone now. The last time we tried it was all I could do to not cry my eyes out and my heart ached for Craig. I keep reminding myself that even though he talks and carries on a conversation with me, his brain is not functioning with his body. The reality is that his body looks whole and perfect. The same as when I get him into the tub and he doesn't know how to sit and when I get him down, he doesn't know how to stand back up again or to lift his leg over the tub. There are just certain things that his brain no longer is able to communicate to his body. When he has gas he can't understand it and says, "Why does that do that, I didn't even touch it—I promise." I just chuckle and say we all do that.

Tonight he was sitting on the couch looking and pulling his stomach and wanted to know where that came from. He reminded me that he couldn't be fat because he is a runner. I told him he was just bloated, that we all get bloated from time to time. Sometimes I don't know how I think to tell him things he needs to hear. And, sometimes I wonder about me. I bought new razors to shave him with now that I've gotten brave enough to leave the electric razor behind. The last two days I've shaved him at night and in the morning and I couldn't believe this new razor did such a lousy job. I went to change the blade tonight thinking it was defective and it was upside down.

I feel sad on some days when Craig thinks I don't like him when I get deep in thought or when I plug away on the computer with this documentation or read the Wall Street Journal. There are times when I just need to be alone with my thoughts or escape from my thoughts, so I read a lot of business type papers and books. I don't know if I have the energy to read a novel and escape that way. I read books but not novels. I did read *The Notebook: A Novel* by Nicholas Sparks and published by Warner Books. It is a short novel about a couple and the woman has Alzheimer's. I just read the article in People magazine that Nancy Reagan wrote about her life with President Reagan. It talks about her being his nurse and her loneliness. I know that feeling well. I know that I have my children and friends, but no one can comprehend your days and nights and what goes on in your mind. This is a person who you thought you would grow old with and he's 54 years old and I'm sure that it's been going on for at least five years now. I know that the weekend I found the lump in my breast and we were in Las Vegas for the half-marathon and we teased Craig when he got lost going to the movies with our friends. That was the beginning and little did I know that the lump in my breast was minor compared to what was ahead of us with Craig's disease. Each has been a learning and a growing experience.

December 14, 1997. *"There is no better exercise for the heart than reaching down and lifting someone up"* — I need to concentrate on balancing my checkbook and paying bills. I have put off paying my property taxes that are now delinquent and I know my bills must be past due. We had a nice time at church today and Taylor, our granddaughter, went with us. He dearly loves his grandchildren. Craig said he even participated in his priesthood group talking about friends and the importance of them. I was proud of him to join in. I think he was proud of himself as well. Santa Claus (my nephew) came by tonight and saw the children and brought presents. He was great. He told the children that as important as Santa Claus is, the most important thing about Christmas is remembering the birth of our Savior, Jesus Christ, and that everytime we see Santa Claus we should remember the true meaning of Christmas, which is Christ. He then joked with each of the children gave them each a present and a little gift of M&M's and then each family got a family gift (game). We then had Christmas cookies, sodas and ice cream cones with sprinkles. The children love playing with each other. We must have spent an hour together with Santa and taking pictures. Even our littlest grandson, Jamison, sat on his lap and to top it off Craig and I sat on each knee. I never know what next Christmas will bring so I try to fill each day with all of the things I should so as to live with no regrets. The main thing now is getting a history written of Craig to give to each of his grandchildren.

Today when we were getting ready for church I cut his chin while I was shaving him and I had a little tissue on it. I told him he could just go sit down and watch television and I would be right there when I got ready. He said he just wanted to stand there and watch me because I was so pretty. I just laughed and he said it's true - you are pretty. He tells me that a lot lately. He also teases me about seeing someone else or liking girls because he said it is six years since we have had sex because he keeps track and he has a great memory. Each time he reminds me about our sex life the number of years change. I tell him it hasn't been that long but he doesn't believe me and rattles on about it for a while. Oh, well. One day at a time.

It was so fun to have the children here tonight laughing and just enjoying each other without anyone rushing and everyone just having a great time. We need to do it more often I suppose. I'll try to do better.

December 15, 1997. *"Who does God's work will get God's pay"* — This seems to be the only thing that keeps me sane anymore. I just sit on the couch and type away while the news shows are on. Craig continually complains that his "butt" is sore and would I help him get in and out of the tub. He said he can't figure out why I can get in and out by myself and he can't. I assure him it is because of the disease and medication. It pacifies him and he lets me help him. He recognizes everyone, remembers relatively well and carries on somewhat of a conversation but yet he can't shave or dress himself. He tries to be independent and will want to put on his own shirt or his own robe or coat and it takes several times but eventually he can do it if you give him enough time. He is still on the "wanting sex" thing and even told his mother today that he was sure I had a boyfriend. This disease is very wicked and I sometimes wish it was something physical and he had his mind and could understand. I hope that when we reach the eternities together that we can laugh at the things I have had to keep from him and figure out and do by myself. I didn't think I would ever be talking to my mother in-law or my children about our sex life, but I have to let them know what is going on because he seems totally uninhibited by whom he says what to and what he says. Steve and Wendy kept him for the day. When Wendy brought him home he went through the same story with her. He did the same thing with Suzanne and a friend. Suzanne called and said it's Dr. Ruth calling. I told Craig that she was giving me a pep talk on sex and he thought that was great.

A friend stopped by tonight and Craig actually went running with him and helped them find their way back because his friend isn't acquainted with the area. Craig has probably gained ten pounds. He is upset at me enough that he wouldn't let me help him get his tights on and he put them on backwards — I didn't tell him and just let him go. I think they only went five miles. He and his wife stayed and ate dinner with us. It is always nice to have people around. It is nice to have people to talk to because he doesn't seem so repetitive and especially when he's upset like he is with me right now. Craig has gone from a 32 to a 36 and they are even a little tight. He doesn't look fat, but I'm just used to him being thin which is the way you stay when you run ten plus miles a day.

I pray for strength and guidance and I want the holidays to be over and spring to come. Oh, well one day at a time.

December 16, 1997. *"Every man goes down to his grave bearing in his hands only that which he has given away"*— Craig spent the morning with his mother and the afternoon with Suzanne and had lunch with Jesse. Craig said Jesse taught him to eat onions and they weren't so bad. Craig didn't like to eat onions or garlic because he didn't want to have bad breath for the public. I got him in the tub tonight before we went to dinner at a friend's and he thought he had gas and had a bowel movement in the tub. I got him out scrubbed the tub and him and then got him back in for a while. He wanted to soak again when we got home from our friends and he did the same thing and it was everywhere this time. I chose not to get him back in this time, just cleaned up and had him go lie down on a heating pad. I know he seems upset and does not know what is going on and to be honest, I don't either. I don't know if he really thinks he's got gas or he just doesn't know what he is doing. We had a lot of laughs at dinner and he is still upset at me enough that he didn't like it when I tried to help him out when he would forget words. Once in a while he would let me help. He let our friend help him with his coat. Our friend actually helped him down the stairs and into the car.

I only wish he didn't have hemorrhoids right now and that would make things a little easier. Between the sex issue and the sore butt I know it's hard for a lot of people. I wish I could give him something to just knock him out at night — for him to not know anything for ten hours and for me just to get a night's sleep. I guess the same for me to knock me out and not think for ten hours.

I realized that we have been in business for ten years this month and I need to have a ten-year anniversary sale and recognize what Craig has accomplished.

December 17, 1997. *"The service we render to others is really the rent we pay for our room on this earth"* — Suzanne took her dad this morning and I worked a half-day and came home. He had another little BM accident and there were a couple of spots on the rug that he had tried to clean up that you could still see, all of his clothes were changed and he was laying on his stomach on the bed. It saddened me and I wanted to cry. I called the surgeon who operated on Craig's hemorrhoids two years ago. He was the same one that performed my Mastectomy. So, I felt that I knew him well enough to call and ask for something. He gave him Cordizone suppositories to use three times a day. I have some cream and thought we could do hot baths in-between times and have him lay on a bed with a heating pad and remain off his feet. Just in case because it is the holidays I made an appointment to go in on Monday. He will see us at 4:00. I thought he was very nice in being so prompt in calling me back and fitting us in to his only day he is working before the holidays. I have certainly got a lot of companions to help me on this journey. I've developed self-confidence and a strength that I didn't know I had before. I've always felt secure, but I'm learning more.

December 18, 1997. *"Life's greatest defeats can be life's greatest victories – if we gained experience and wisdom from them"* — Our 32nd anniversary. I bought myself a pair of silver earrings. They have taken on new meaning since he gave me the exact pair two years in a row. I did not remind Craig of the significance of the day. Bill, Dave and Garth took Craig to lunch at a buffet style restaurant today. They all stood in the line got their food, went back to the table and realized Craig wasn't there. Bill went to locate him and he was sitting in another booth arguing with two women. They told him that was their booth and he said it wasn't because he was there with his friends. They asked him where they were and he told them they were coming. The manager joined in and Bill found him. He told Craig they decided to go to another table and then after Craig got up to leave explained to the ladies and the manager. All was forgiven. Craig never knew he was on the wrong side of the restaurant. I believe at the time only Bill knew and understood the severity of Craig's disease. The three of them gave him a Christmas present. It was a box with three rolls of quarters (for golf they would bet quarters) and some golf balls. He showed me when he got home and cried that he had such wonderful friends. He reminded himself that it wasn't nice what he said about one friend. I asked what it was and he said that if he had been in the Donner party they could have survived for an extra week on one of his thighs. We laughed.

December 19, 1997. *"May I take time to be of service to others"* — Well, I'm home from work again. Steve stopped by to visit and show his dad his new truck. Craig is so proud of his children. Suzanne checks on her dad everyday or with me to see what needs to be done and Steve calls him every night to talk to him. I'm going to stay home from the store tomorrow as well and Sunday not have Craig go to church. Monday will be here and hopefully the doctor can do something for him. His hemorrhoids do look terrible. I'm at a loss as to know what else to do. I feel like I just want to sit in a room somewhere and not listen, do or see. Actually, what it amounts to is that I continue to wish each day away.

December 21, 1997. *"To have a good friend is one of the highest delights of life, to be a good friend is one of the noblest and most difficult undertakings"* — I worked at the store for three hours yesterday just to get away and escape reality. I've decided that you have to do that and not feel guilty. It is what gets you through each day. Our neighbor came down and stayed with Craig and gave him his pill and dinner at 5:00. I try to be consistent with medication times. He seems less anxious. Our friends, Richard and Jan, stopped by with a Christmas gift and visited for a while. Friends are true treasures – gifts from God. Richard's mother has Alzheimer's and they take turns staying with her. They understand what I am going through. I went to the first part of church and had Craig stay home. He got up and had a nice dinner and then got in the tub again and we did the suppositories and the rest. I went to work for an hour but Craig thinks I just ran to the store. He is sometimes possessive of me and where and how I spend my time. He's going to spend the morning with his mother tomorrow and then have lunch with Bob and Richard. It will be fun for him to get out with friends. These lunches are not for much longer and I'm sure it will have a lasting impact on these friends that spend this time with him. They will have some fond memories of having helped a friend — both Craig and me.

Craig is becoming more scattered with his speech and thoughts and I'm filling in the blanks more. The last two days he seems to not know his way around the house as much or gets more twisted around. His sister called this morning and said he seems so much more spiritual.

I saw a neighbor at church and talked to her about the cost of resthomes. Her husband died of Parkinson's. She said that one cost $3,000 a month. I'm more astounded everyday by what I learn of costs. I don't know how the average person continues to stay afloat when they are as young as we are. I am continually amazed that nothing is covered with this disease or any form of dementia.

I received a gift today from my good friend in Boston and from a gentleman I work for and his sweet wife. All very good friends. I think I will unwrap my gifts from my friends on Christmas Eve so that on Christmas morning I will unwrap my slippers just as Craig will. He's never mentioned buying gifts or asked what we have for anyone. So, I don't know what he is even thinking about. Mostly I guess we'll get tomorrow's doctor appointment over with then Tuesday, then Christmas and then we are on the downhill slide into spring and summer. Then I dare let him run on his own if he chooses to. I don't dare let him go running now by himself because of the low temperatures, even with his necklace that says he is memory impaired. It frightens me for anyone to be lost in cold weather. I hope my little sister will go to Salt Lake with us on Tuesday so that we can have Christmas lunch together. It's been a long time since I've seen her. I think of her often with all the little things she has done to help me around the house. There are little touches of her everywhere.

December 22, 1997. *"Life only gives you time and space, it's up to you to fill it"* — Craig and I went to the surgeon's today to have his hemorrhoids checked. He wants us to have his prostate checked and said that there shouldn't be that much blood because the hemorrhoids are actually looking better. He wants me to continue the suppositories for another week and then get back with him. Oh, it just seems like there is always one more thing. I guess after Alzheimer's we could handle almost anything. I tell myself that, and I usually believe myself. I plunk away each night and it seems to bring me some peace and I wish I could sit here and plunk away forever. It seems like I keep putting things off until the last minute and know that I can't put it off any longer. Maybe there is some depression — I don't know. I like night times when we go to bed and I like first thing in the morning when I sit all by myself in the quiet and dark of the early morning. A nephew stopped by last night to visit. I had gone to bed early with Craig (8:00) and our daughter came in and woke me up and it startled me. I guess I was more tired than I thought. We had a cup of hot chocolate together and he offered to help me however he could.

December 23, 1997. *Life is like a mirror, give to the world the best you have and the best will come back to you"* — I went to work for just a little bit to check in and check out. I'm going to be lost after the holidays when I need to be at work each morning at a set time and I'll need to stay for an entire day. I'm feeling the need to take responsibility for Craig's care each day while I can still keep him at home. We went to the Pharmacology Research Center today. They felt like Craig was declining too, but Craig seemed less anxious than the last time. We haven't been there in three months and we don't go back until mid-April. Our participation in the study ends after that time, but we can continue if we want. The doctor did say today that he doesn't note much change in Craig with the medication as he does in some of the older patients that he sees. He said that it does proceed at a much faster pace in younger people such as Craig. He said, "I wish I could say where I see him next June, but none of us know. It is a day-by-day thing." Craig seems still to be obsessed with sex saying that I don't like him anymore. It makes me feel sad, but I also know it's not Craig. His weight was 186 today and last May he weighed in at 164. I told the doctor that we had graduated to a 36-waist size and he said a lot of people lose weight. I'm sure Craig will too one day as his eating changes. Right now he seems to want to eat every few hours saying it makes him feel better. I don't even know what I think about anymore. I used to enjoy getting up and watching the early morning news. Now, I get up and sit in the quiet in my own little corner and don't even turn the television on and wait for Craig to get up and tell me he needs food. If it is too early I tell him he needs to go back to bed for a while and he says, "I knew you were going to tell me that." While I have the luxury of not going to work until 10:00 I just let him sleep. We stopped at a store today to pick up a little gift and he walked so far behind me and so slow that I almost lost him. I had him wear his necklace that I'm grateful for. It frightened me for a minute and I don't know what was going through his mind. He doesn't like to hold my hand or have me help him. I think it is his independence taken away, much like when I try to help him with his jacket and he wants to do it by himself. I find that lately I have a harder time concentrating on things I need to do at work or for the store or anything. It's like I just want to hop off somewhere and not think about anything. Yet, I enjoy being at work and escaping from the day-to-day of being a Caregiver. By escaping – I mean that it is an overwhelming feeling that you are losing your best friend and your spouse. The doctor at the clinic talked about trying Day Care again and also mentioned talking to the BYU Psychological Clinic to see if they would be interested in setting up a program much like the Family Living department does for child care. I thought that was an interesting concept. I think I will talk to our friend at the BYU Comprehensive Clinic and get his thoughts on it. It might be something that could help someone in the future, just not Craig. That is one of the things that I could do as I pursue avenues to help others, in particular younger Alzheimer patients. Students could chart the decline of the patients in the daycare program like you would a child in a daycare program.

December 25, 1997. *"Christmas is a time to remember timeless stories from days of yore, a time to ponder what's ahead, a time to open another door"* — Craig slept until almost 8:30 this morning. He says his butt still hurts and we ate, showered and dressed and went over to Suzanne & Stephen's to see the children and Craig had pancakes with them. We then went to Steve and Wendy's for lunch and took them their gifts and watched Taylor and Madison unwrap the last of their presents. Craig always has fun watching them. We went over to Suzanne's last night for Christmas dinner. We had turkey, and it is always good to be around others. Craig always seems more together and happier around more people, or I should say family and/or close friends. We unwrapped our slippers this morning and that was our Christmas from Santa. Craig got a new shirt and jacket with Steve's Good Neighbor logo and a quilt from Suzanne that the children drew pictures on. These were special gifts to Craig. I got a book on

"Counting My Blessings" (of which I know I have many) and a CD "You'll Never Walk Alone" (I won't). I know how many people walk with me every day both in words and deeds. I feel more alone each day and overwhelmed with Craig's disease. Or, perhaps it isn't Craig, but that I'm overwhelmed with decisions about where I am headed myself alone. It's time-consuming knowing what I need to do.

We had a wonderful day with the children. Craig stayed with Steve. Wendy and I took the girls to a movie. It was nice to get out. Steve fixed his dad some spaghetti before we got back. I forgot to remind him of his dad's eating habits. He thinks he needs to eat constantly or he'll get sick (or he forgets he's eaten).

Another interesting tidbit is that Craig has always been meticulous with his clothes and the minute we come in the house he takes his coat off and just drops it on the floor. And, when he takes his clothes off to get in the tub and get ready for bed, same thing. He just drops them on the floor wherever he is standing. He's like a toddler.

Our neighbors, Richard and Mary Ann, came down tonight and put a new shower hose/head on for him. That will be wonderful to help me shower him. He won't have to move and I can move the hose head around. It will be safer and easier for both of us. They have been very good to Craig and very helpful to me.

December 27, 1997. *"Love makes one richer than a mountain of gold"* — I spent the day home with Craig and then put a video in for him and worked at the store from 4:00-6:00. He's fine by himself for a few hours as long as he has anti-depressants regularly with food and drink. He seems more confused these past few days. Today he asked me if we lived together in the same house. Yet, he calls me by name and says what he needs to do and then says I'm confused - I don't know where I'm at. When he needs to go to the bathroom he starts undressing before he gets there. I have to watch him when we are at someone's home or if we go to a restaurant. He seems frightened enough at the thought of going to a public restroom that he doesn't go until we get home. He gets confused about getting in the car and where the handle is to get in. He frightens me by where he holds his hand on the roof of the car at getting himself into the car that I now hold the door until I know his hands, and feet are in and then I close the door. He doesn't know how to get himself out of the car most times. I remember once driving along the canyon road and he saw somebody he knew and he went to open the door to yell at them because he didn't know how to get the window down. I now do the childproof locks. Sometimes when we see someone he knows he will knock on the window and yell at them like they can hear him. I just respond back to him by saying I don't think they heard you. Pretty much I don't say whom I see or call anything to his attention while we are in the car. I try to keep conversation to a minimum. He likes listening to soft music with no words so we keep a CD in the car that he listens to. One of the tunes he likes to repeat is *Softly As I Leave You*. He cries and asks if we can hear it again.

Some days I feel like a hermit as I sit here alone plugging away with my thoughts. I know that people want to know about Craig, but they also don't know what to say or even to ask, and I never know quite what to say. I've tried to be very honest with people and let them know that this is a horrible disease. It's the only way to educate people. I feel like friends and family tend to keep at a distance. I watch out for Craig like I'm his parent. Craig is up and down so much and he takes all of my time and attention during my waking and sleeping hours. There are no free hours.

December 29, 1997. *"No one has ever injured his eyesight by looking on the bright side of their journey"* — Susie, my sister, picked Craig up at 10:00 today and they met his friend Jesse for breakfast. Susie and Craig then went to Salt Lake to visit my other two sisters. They even went to a show, but I'm still trying to decide what they saw. Craig seems to be upset with me a lot and he'll talk with other people and try to avoid me. As I try to help him dress or fill in the blanks when he's talking he doesn't like it. Craig has always been a happy and kind person but now he gets upset periodically. I know they say or I've read that people get mean and I've been asked that a lot. So, I guess if this is as mean as he gets I need to be okay with that. It's just that I know how much effort it takes for me each day and it's wearing. I think I have bags under my eyes every day. As I said before he likes to get in the tub every night. If it makes him feel good I'm okay with whatever. I've noticed the last few nights that when he asks if he can get in the tub, he gets confused and calls it pud. He told Susie he is upset at me and that I don't want anything to do with him. This is probably the beginning of the hard times ahead. We may end up at day-care sooner than I think because I don't think Suzanne will be able to cope with the sex conversations daily. Craig's slipping.

December 31, 1997. *"That which we learn pleasantly, we retain"* — Well, here it is the last day of 1997. The years just seem to be tumbling by faster and faster. Craig just got out of the tub again and said his butt is feeling better because his mother put hot packs on him today and that the reason it gets sore is because he has to keep going to the bathroom. He dried off and dressed himself tonight. I know that his shorts are on backwards and I don't know about the top. I didn't see it because he put his own robe on even though it probably took 5-6 minutes. I hope to be able to go to work tomorrow for awhile. I try to monitor the phone conversations with friends to only say positive, short comments. I do most of my calls when I get Craig in bed or from my cell phone. Not only do you feel like you are in life alone, but you feel like your words and actions are monitored. To a degree they are, so you watch what you say and do around them. He is afraid to go to bed alone so I always go with him, get him to sleep and then quietly get back up and write in the quiet hours of my aloneness.

I so miss being able to put my arms around him, give him hugs and tell him how much I love him and have him respond back. I'm watching "Casablanca" by myself on New Year's Eve.

January 1, 1998. *"It is more important to know where we are going than to get there quickly"* — The first day of the New Year. Craig went running at 9:00 with our neighbor. They ran to the temple and back. Craig came back and soaked in the tub because of his sore butt. It makes people uncomfortable when he talks about his hemorrhoids but they laugh. Our neighbor came and sat with him for a couple of hours and I went to work and on a couple of errands. I came back and got lunch for him and decided to go to Salt Lake and get me some new shoes. I treated myself to shoes and earrings. Last year I bought me some silver earrings from Craig and they were clip on instead of pierced. I sometimes wonder where my brain is. I do things without thinking. We had meat pies when I got home around 4:00. At 6:00 he was breathing hard and heavy and saying he needed food and where was I. I tried to tell him he just ate an hour ago and he just got upset at me and told me he ought to know when he's hungry. He sat and breathed so fast and hard that I thought he was going to hyperventilate before I got the food to him. It's like some little kid throwing a tantrum and you're trying to appease him, but he isn't a little kid and he doesn't know he's doing it. Now it's almost 8:00 and he wants to know when it is time to go to bed and yet he won't go until I go. Steve called tonight to say "hi" and Craig wants to go to lunch with him and visit. I called Steve back to tell him to be prepared to talk about our sex life or lack of and Steve said oh, brother, I hope you are kidding – one thing a person doesn't want to talk about is his parents' sex life. I told him I didn't think he had a choice, and to remember Dad is sick and just listen and agree to whatever is said. Steve did as he was asked and it was tough duty. Wendy brought him home and he had the same conversation with her. Steve called and said please don't make us do that again. I could only hope. I'll also be glad when this phase of "sexual" fascination is over. Craig is beyond caring or knowing about the store anymore. It would definitely be a transition to have it be gone since it has been a part of my life for the past ten years as well as Craig's.

January 3, 1998. *"May wisdom, determination and perseverance increase all my days"* — Today we started out early getting Craig ready to go run with the race team. We picked up our neighbor at 7:45 a.m. and he even kept up with the race team for the 10 miles they ran. They all came back to the store for bagels and juice. It's always fun to visit with Craig's running friends. They are kind and dedicated friends. They offered to take turns picking Craig up to run and just take him at nights for a few hours to give me a break. I feel unbelievably blessed with his friends, or I should say our friends. Bob and Richard are going to pick him up at 6:30 tomorrow morning, run and then go to breakfast before church. It's early, but it will also give me two hours to myself and then we'll just be late for church.

Craig went to his mother's today while I went to work for a few hours, and then he went to Suzanne's and came home to take a nap he said. He must have gone to the bathroom and taken his shorts off. He was going to the bathroom after I came home and his jeans were on the floor and he didn't have any underclothes on and his shoes were not tied. I had asked Suzanne to pick me up some milk today at the store and she sent it home with Craig to put it in the fridge. We couldn't find it tonight and looked everywhere for it. We finally found it in the freezer. We had a good laugh. I don't know if he thought it was funny or not. He seems to be a lot more scattered. I think we are both physically exhausted tonight. It was a long day.

January 4, 1998. *"I will make time for myself"* — I got up at 5:30 this morning and sat in the quiet for 30 minutes before I woke Craig up to eat a bowl of cereal and get dressed to go run with Bob and Richard. I wanted to shave him before he ran so that when they brought him home at 8:30 he could shower and get dressed to go to church. And, since I have to help him with these things it seems to take longer because he so wants to do it alone. Tonight he wanted some toast while we watched *60 Minutes*. He calls it "doase" or "doast" — I can't understand him exactly. Sometimes it is so funny some of the things that he says that I want to laugh. He told me today that I shouldn't have told him that it's okay to have gas because that makes you need to "poop" and he shouldn't be doing that. Then he worries that he doesn't flush the toilet enough. He holds the handle down until all of the water is gone. I've also noticed how much he shuffles instead of actually picking up his feet to walk especially when he is going to the bathroom. The minute we come in from outside he throws his coat off and on the floor.

I've decided that as a New Year's resolution to help me I need to do one good deed a day - actually go out of my way to do something nice or good for someone. These next three days will be very interesting since I need to be to work at an early hour and work until 5 or 6:00 each day. I guess I will ask Suzanne and see if she will keep him all day those three days and then ask Steve to take him to lunch each day.

January 6, 1998. *"Live so you don't regret the things you've done"* — I had a good talk with Suzanne tonight. She talked to her dad about sex and said it isn't something that you talk to your children, mother, friends and others about. It should be something that only you and your spouse talk about. She promised that she would talk to her mom for him. She told him that love meant more than sex and that she knew mom loved him very much because she shaved, showered, bathed and dressed him every day and got all of his meals and cleaned up after him. He agreed and when he came home he said, "I'm sorry." I knew what he meant and I said, thank you. I want to just be able to put my arms around him and say how much I love him but I have a hard time holding him and not sobbing. And, I know I can't do that. This is so hard. You feel like you are in a catch-22 situation. Tonight Suzanne admitted that she, too, has thought about death being sweet. Then she said that if dad can handle it everyday that we should be able to handle it as well. I know we are each growing and learning each day. Today he had several near misses with bowel movement accidents. There are dirty jeans, towels and underpants in the hamper. I think tomorrow morning I am going to buy some Depends. It will be interesting to see if he is aware as I try them. He is scheduled for a scope of his colon on Friday. It is same-day surgery. Thursday is a liquid only day with laxatives twice per day. This should be an interesting day as well as Friday morning until I get him there. I hope the Depends will come in handy on that day as well. Each night as I plug away on the computer he asks what I am doing. I just remind him that I am working for a minute. He thinks I am married to my work. Oh, if he only had an inkling, I wonder what he would do or if he had known or understood how this would be playing out now. I remind myself I never want to know. I couldn't imagine it any other way than the way we are doing it. Right now he seems obsessed with that it isn't normal that you 'poop'. I told him everyone does and he doesn't believe me. Oh, well.

January 7, 1998. *"Don't worry be happy" — (This was Craig's favorite saying – he used it the day he opened the store)* We just got back from dinner with Mike and Linda. They are good friends. Craig wanted to know if they had children. (Their son is 32) He told them about his butt and how I burned it and how he worried about my 'smarts' and how they dealt with me at work. We were all laughing. I think they had a great time as well. Linda said she didn't remember when she laughed so much. Craig says things and uses his hands so much to talk that you think you're going to get your eyes poked out. I spaced off making two calls that I was supposed to make. Between three days of meetings and preparing and cleaning up from them is exhausting. I believe in my heart that Craig is fine and that all of the blood was because of his hemorrhoids. The worst part is telling the doctor that it was my fault that he has a burn on each cheek from the heating pad. I can't believe he didn't feel it being too hot. He seems to be possessive of me when I get home from work. If I have to go the store he will be hyperventilating when I get home and he will tell me he needs food. I'll give him a little Gatorade and a couple of crackers then he seems fine.

January 8, 1998. *"Walk with gratitude towards Him"* — I told Craig about his liquid diet this morning when he woke up. He wasn't thrilled, but accepted. I've fed him Jell-O, Gatorade, juices and broth. He took the first dose of an oral laxative. I bought Depends just in case. I've asked him to watch television in the bedroom just across from the bathroom so he'll be close. He can then 'surf' as he calls it with the television remote. They told me that he could have his sleeping pill tonight which is a good thing. I feel like I am just existing lately. As Craig goes in for the colonoscopy tomorrow I've thought about all sorts of things. I've heard wonderful things about the doctor who is doing the procedure. I look forward to meeting him.

January 9, 1998. *"Look out for the tongue, it is in a wet place and may slip"* — I talked to the Alzheimer's Association. I've been soliciting donations for a dinner/fund-raiser for Alzheimer's. Suzanne and Wendy said they would go with me. It's a $75 a plate dinner and I want to be able to meet the people I should know that affects what is going on in my life with Craig. I want to be involved with the Alzheimer's Association. We are caught between two worlds of young and old – real and unreal. We made it through the day. The laxatives weren't so bad and we had no accidents. He did better without solid food than I had anticipated. It's 9:00 and he got in a hot tub and went to bed. I told him I needed to sleep in the other bed so I could sleep and wake up to the alarm.

January 10, 1998. *"Time, a most precious gift, take advantage of every minute"* — Another night. Craig is upset again. It's wearing. He wanted to say hi to two friends at the store before he went to his mother's and two other friends were at the store. He went and had an Oreo shake with them. A friend from Salt Lake came down to bring us the '98 race schedule. He went down to talk to Craig. Another friend came in to pick up a race form and went down as well. He had a nice visit with everyone. He spent the afternoon at his mother's. He was anxious to come home even though he isn't thrilled lately when he sees me. He just wants to come home. The minute he gets into the car he says he's got to go home and use the bathroom, he didn't like the food very well and he's got to have something to eat. I made him some hot chocolate and toast with peanut butter and jelly. He wanted to watch television in the other room. He doesn't like it when I type on the computer. He's becoming more possessive of my time and me. When I go to the store to work on Saturday he reminds me that I'm not supposed to do that anymore. I think this week I truly came to grips with the thought of caring for him like a child. It is wearing both physically and emotionally. I feel I exist day-to-day. Talking is more charades, and one-on-one, it's hard. When there are more people involved it's not so hard to play charades. It makes it more of a game. Craig has so many wonderful friends that want to help. I don't know how to have them help except just pick him up and take him to lunch or run. I know they are both hard. As nice as it is to have his friends pick him up on Sunday's it, too, is hard. I have to wake him up early, shave and dress him to be ready. I value the hour and a half he is gone to play catch-up with myself. That's always gratifying. I did get the January Race Team Newsletter off today. There are a lot of things I need to do to update myself with the store, order procedures and just overall things.

January 11, 1998. *"Education is learning the rules and experience is learning the exceptions"* — Today was the early run with Craig's friends: Bob, Ed and Richard. Bob and Richard both showed up to pick him up at 6:50 a.m. They have to help him navigate the stair on the front porch, into the truck and fasten his seatbelt for him. They are so kind to Craig. Ed brings him home. Craig said there were eight running this morning. I have no idea who the others were or if there were eight. He needed to eat again and then was slow to shower and dress. We only went to the last half of church. He's more confused when we get to the church as to where we go. He's also very snappy with me lately. I think I am feeling at an all-time low. I just want to be able to go to a movie or run away from everything for a few days. I went to the store and bought a family in need some groceries, dropped them off on their porch and that was my good deed for the day. It's not often I am able to do this. It makes me feel good to share or do some small gesture for someone. I'm sure Craig's friends must have this same good feeling. When I returned home after being gone for less than an hour he snapped he had to have 'roughage' I'm sick. I never know what roughage is and since I knew we would be eating dinner in two hours I gave him a bowl of cereal with a banana sliced on it. I think maybe I'm just exhausted with the ordeal of the last three days. I keep thinking I will get a good book but I'm always too scattered to concentrate on reading a novel. I enjoy keeping busy but I have a hard time concentrating to read. I just need to go to work and plow into it. I've got to get myself organized since we're moving offices. I need to be a better friend to people around me. I need to be a better friend to myself. I get in my own little world and don't let anyone in. It's not healthy. Craig's disease is taking a toll of my 'letting my light shine' desire or attitude. Craig as he goes to the bathroom just stares into the toilet bowl. I have to remind him to turn around. When he flushes it he holds it down for what seems forever. Then he flushes three to four times. I believe he thinks that all the water in the toilet bowl is his own urine or 'pee' as he calls it lately. A few times I've noticed he says he needs to tinkle.

January 12, 1998. *"Discover wisdom"* — Craig woke up at 6:30 today. He went to bed at 8:15 though. I'm always exhausted myself so I don't even care. It's nice to have quiet. Listening to him to talk to Jesse tonight was exhausting. He was so repetitive and kept asking questions. The friends that still talk to him and take him places are so wonderful. He does seem better when he talks to them and he seems upbeat instead of down like he is with me lately. I try very hard to always be happy and upbeat around him like there is nothing out of the ordinary. I think I act like everything is 'normal'. Suzanne kept him today. She read a book on 'toileting' to him. He said how the food goes to your esophagus and then stomach so he shouldn't have to go to the toilet right after he eats like he thinks he does. She said he wanted to keep snacking and then rest. He was asleep when I got home. He got up, used the bathroom and said he needed to eat. He had snacks at Suzanne's, ate lunch at his mother's and had somehow managed to eat a bunch of bananas I had at home (at least 10). I don't know how he can consume that many.

January 13, 1998. *"Enjoy the moment"* — I'm alone for an hour while Craig is running with Debbie and her husband Ron at the BYU track. I am so appreciative of Craig's friends that take him. Craig and I seem to talk less when he appears upset. He did thank me tonight when I gave him two Tylenol's for his headache, which seem to be more frequent. I think in the 35 minutes we were waiting for them to pick him up to run he said he had to use the bathroom eight times. Each time he went to unzip his jacket and I would remind him that he just needed to pull his pants down. Most times he understood. Today when I picked him up from his mother's, she told him as we left to be a nice husband and he said, "I don't think that's possible." She said she talked to him today and told him that men and women are different. I believe his mother now understands the depth of how far and how fast he is failing. When Craig was first diagnosed she had a hard time believing and told me she wanted a third opinion and she didn't want it to be mine. I'm sure it was extremely hard for a mother to realize that such a healthy, young son could have a terminal disease such as Alzheimer's. Craig this morning did not know his sister when I mentioned her name. He questioned me about her all the way to his mother's this morning. When the phone rings he wants to know who it is and what they want. He's like a monitor. This is a disease where you sometimes wish your life away. First, I wished I could sell the store and get my own life in order and then do the things I need to get his ready. I want to review where we are and be there for Craig. He likes things simple and plain. I want him to be free and running with the angels and out of this hell that he must be in as well. I love being able to take care of him and serve him and it is going to be a mixed bag when he is able to go home to be with his Heavenly Father.

January 14, 1998. *"Smile, it's contagious"* — I woke up early after a very sleepless night. I got up and made myself some hot chocolate and ate cake in the dark in my little corner with my heating pad. I felt myself spilling the cake and so I finally got a flashlight to help me see the cake. I never want to turn the lights on and wake Craig up. I've thought more than ever today after listening to a song by Alabama entitled "An Angel Amongst Us" that Craig has been the angel in our life, and I am learning along with so many others what life is and what it is about. It doesn't matter what our position in life, the dollars in the bank or where we live but, what is in our heart and what we do to reach out to others...how we treat our fellow brothers and sisters. Craig definitely enriched my life and I hope I can pass that richness on. He taught me so much. I learn patience with him in trying to understand. Tonight when I finally said I knew what he was talking about when I didn't he told me never to lie because Heavenly Father doesn't like me when I lie. So now I just say I don't know. He is complaining of his headache tonight and keeps wanting me to help him go to the bathroom. I finally told him to just lay down and try to relax and maybe his head will feel better. I wish I knew what was going on when he tells me his head is going to blow off. I know that he is eating well and resting well. This is a wicked illness and I truly believe that anything physical has got to be better. He is becoming more agitated with me when I try to fill in the blanks when he is telling people something or if I try to give my opinion. I've decided it's better not to say anything at all. I pray for God to help me be strong. I've decided we have to continue to laugh. I've decided he must have had a wonderful time on the business trips he's been on with Novations and myself because he talks about it to others frequently. He seems to be more confused with more things and I find myself pointing all the time even though it makes him more agitated. In the mornings I point to the toilet forever to have him sit there so I can shave him. I know that it is important to just focus on each day and live day-to-day. I continually pray that I might have strength. I am not in this alone. Jesse took him to lunch today and he had a good time but said the food was "shitty" — he says that about a lot of food that he eats when he is away from me. I don't know what he considers good anymore. I don't think he liked the chili we had tonight until I told him Kathy made it especially for him. Then, he said it was the "best stuff I ever ate." I need to go turn down the bed and check on him and get him to bed for the night. I think I have a headache myself tonight. I think Sunday's are my favorite day, too, now just so that I don't need to take Craig anywhere.

January 15, 1998. *"Never give up"* — Craig spent the day with his sister. I think he enjoyed himself and he wanted to call her tonight to say thank you because she wasn't there when I picked him up. Her son is great with Craig and always gives him a hug. We had dinner tonight with an old school friend. It was an interesting night. Craig had a hard time finding words and remembering names and when he uses his hands his fingers are right in your face. He even gets a little upset with me in front of people now because he is so anxious about not remembering. He still knows a lot because as you go to help him with his coat he wants to do it himself. But, when you are in a restaurant it is hard because he knocks things off the table and people are so close I think he's going to hit someone. I've decided it's easier to eat at home just the two of us. There is less stress. I've been doing spreadsheets for the store tonight. We need to order for spring '98 and tomorrow we meet with the shoe rep to order shoes for fall of '98. I have a peace about me that I haven't had in a while. I really believe everything will be okay long term. And, the store seems to be doing okay.

January 16, 1998. *"Life is a test without an instruction manual"* — We ordered summer shoes today. Steve, Terry and I did the ordering. I tell Craig all ordering is done on the phone now. I took Craig down there when Wayne was through with everyone to visit with him. I know it was hard for Wayne but there is still that part of me that wants to do the things I know have always made him happy. I have got to soon realize that this isn't Craig anymore. It did make him happy. They had a great visit. It made me feel good that he and Craig were able to spend 30 minutes of quality time together. He got upset at me tonight when I said I wasn't going to fix him anything else to eat that it was time to go to bed. He swore, threw his robe and slammed the bedroom door so hard that I thought it would break. This is so unlike Craig. He has always been so soft and gentle.

January 17, 1998. *"There are no guarantees in life"* — I spent the morning with Craig and we watched Emily for an hour. We had lunch together and then I took Craig to his mother's while I went to the store to work for the afternoon. She didn't know what it was like to have him out of his element at the grocery store. First, he had a hard time with her driving in the dark and not wearing seat belts. Then in the store just walking around had to be very hard for her and I know it's hard for Craig. She called Suzanne after she got home and told her she thought she was about to have a nervous breakdown taking him to the store. I think people don't comprehend until they take him for a period of time and take him out of his element. His mother dropped him off at Suzanne's and she brought him home, turned on the lights and gave him a sandwich. I came home, put his pants on and went to Linda's to visit for a while. I couldn't help but laugh when he was telling me about his mother and the store. I know how sad it is, but just to listen to him was hilarious. I've decided it's easier for me to have him at home and not go anywhere as well. Life is more tolerable. I am so tired tonight. I just want to escape reality for one day. No one is used to Craig ever being upset with me or really anyone so it's hard at first then you have to realize that this isn't Craig. I'm exhausted tonight and am anxious for Craig to go with his friends in the morning.

January 18, 1998. *"Everyone faces struggles"* — It has been quite a day. I woke up at 2:00 and took two Advil for a migraine and went back to bed. I woke up at 5:15 to the sound of the alarm to get Craig up, fed and dressed to go run with Bob, Richard and Ed. He didn't understand that I didn't feel well. I went back to bed after he left and slept until he got home. I was too sick to go to church. I don't know how he got his running clothes off and his robe on. I slept the day away on the couch and ordered a pizza for our lunch and we ate it for dinner as well. We talked to Su tonight for a minute and she was laughing as Craig was talking to her and trying to have her figure out with my help who or what he was talking about. He thinks because phones allow us to talk to people away that they can see what we can see. He was showing her a picture of people she might know. She said she loved and admired me and asked if it was like this all the time. His dad left a poem on the table yesterday with a note. The majority of people unless they are around him for a period of time still do not realize the extent of his disease. It takes some people longer to understand the extent of it. I sometimes lose patience with people and their inability to see or understand the depth and scope of this disease. People think I exaggerate Craig's decline. Why a person would want to do that I have no idea.

January 19, 1998. *"Be grateful for each new day, a new beginning"* — The end of another day. It was Martin Luther King Day so it was a day with school out and other holidays. I had an eye appointment and didn't go to work until later. I found out that my eyes, for being those of an almost 55-year-old, are almost 20-20. My one eye fails a little close and the other a little further away so they compensate each other. So, I guess I won't get any glasses. The person that checked my eyes knew Craig and I ended up crying more than I didn't. I try to stay strong most of the time and feel blessed. I talked to Su tonight to give her a little encouragement to let the bad thoughts go. It's hard to be a caregiver and have happy thoughts all the time. Her mother has Parkinson and she is the full-time caregiver. I couldn't imagine if I didn't get a break. It completely wears you out with filling in the blanks, repetitiveness and all the one-on-one. Steve calls each night to check on his dad. Suzanne called to ask him to talk to her because she rushed him when he was talking to her and Emily was crying. She is very thoughtful of his feelings even though she understands the disease.

January 20, 1998. *"Let your light shine that others may seek it"* — Craig stayed with his mother today — all day. I believe she was ready for me when I got home. My heart aches for her as well. It's got to be heartbreaking for her as his mother to see her son who was always the epitome of health. None of us expect to tend our grown children. Our children are caring for both of their parents. Steve sent me flowers today telling me of his love. He said when he woke up this morning he just wanted to do something special for me. He's very thoughtful and kind. Craig's disease is hard on all of us. Alex tonight asked if I was going to be 55 on my birthday and was I old. I told him I feel young but I am going to be 55. I told Suzanne if I was wealthy I would have a face-lift and she just laughed (I was kidding). I don't know who I want to look young for when it's me, my children and my grandchildren and none of us care if I grow old and have wrinkles. Craig went running with Karen, Debbie and Jeannie of the race team tonight at the BYU track. They are great to pick him up and guide him around. They shield him around the corners and then he does pretty good except his 22 pounds he's gained he gets hot. Of course he has no idea of the extra weight. He does talk about his head hurting a lot and tonight when he got home I had a hot tub ready and shampooed his hair, gave him some hot chocolate to relax him. I'm hoping that he'll sleep well tonight and not wake up at all. He complains about his eyes and not seeing well too. I know that he couldn't read an eye chart and that perhaps since it's been a year when he had the Radiokeratonomy done it may need to be fine tuned but that's not an option. I'm hoping that his vision stays well enough to see him through to graduation. He truly is becoming more confused every day. He gets quite agitated when I plunk away on this laptop. He wanted to go watch television in the other room. I went in and turned it on for him and he said I want to tell you that I think you're a good friend but not a good wife. I know this is not Craig talking and that he is referring to sex only. I wish I could talk to him and explain things while he is somewhat able to comprehend, but I can't because he doesn't understand. It's better that I just swallow hard when he tells me these things. As he sat in the tub tonight he kept telling me all the yellow that he saw was pee. There was no yellow and I have no idea if he urinated in the bath water or not.

January 21, 1998. *"We learn from our experiences"* — Suzanne tended her dad today and Jesse took him to lunch. When he asked where he was going today I told him Suzanne's and it took him a while to figure out who she was when I told him she was our daughter. I also called Jesse to thank him in advance. He said he just remembers that he is one of my companions on this journey we're on. Actually, they know that it is not like Craig either and that it isn't him anymore. We've lost him. It's not even the shell of Craig. Today when I came home he found a bag of cookies and he ate one bite out of at least eight and then there were a couple of bites out of an apple and 3 bananas that he ate. He said he was afraid of Suzanne today. She was blunt with him about not eating or telling him that he can't be hungry because he just ate and when I'm blunt with him he gives me the finger or just becomes upset with me. He has started to just moan when he goes to the bathroom. He just sits on the toilet and moans and tells me he needs help. He actually urinated on the rug when he got out of the tub tonight. The last two nights he's been very unstable about where his feet go to get out of the tub. I have a hard time at nights anymore while we watch television. He rattles on and on and is more repetitive than ever. It's almost a relief when he goes to the other room to watch television and "flip." I've noticed when he goes to the bathroom he pulls a lot of toilet tissue off and leaves little "wads" of tissue on the floor in the bathroom and hallway. He always wants me to look in the toilet and tell him everything is okay. He likes to chew gum a lot lately too. I don't trust him with it because he spits it out anywhere. I don't buy it any more. The last time I found it in the dirty clothes hamper. He just spit it out there. He thinks he needs to "pee" every 10-15 minutes when we're watching television at night. I leave the lights on and tell him he can go by himself. He becomes obsessed with the phone as well. He wants to know who it is and what they want. I have no idea what is going on in the bathroom, but the toilet has flushed at least four times in the last five minutes. He forgets that he's gone to the bathroom just like he forgets he's eaten. He's pretty good about washing his hands after he uses the bathroom but he forgets how to dry his hands and just rubs them on his pants.

January 22, 1998. *"Reach out to others"* — He spent the day with his mother. I didn't shave him very well today. He was angry and wouldn't hold his head up. He told me I'm not only not a good wife, but I'm not a good friend anymore either. I told him I still thought of him as a good friend. I hope I pass my test soon. One of the race team members, Karen, picked him up at 4:15 today to go run the trails, let him eat dinner with her family and then the two of them are going to Lehi to have Paul give them a rub-down. I had a bubble bath, washed my hair, pressed clothes for work, read and am now just typing away. It's very quiet. She said they wouldn't be home until 9:00. I treated myself to a chocolate eclair as well. I feel totally consumed with the day-to-day of everything. I've decided that it would be wonderful for Craig to be able to leave this early existence while his grandchildren remember him as a healthy and vital person who knew them. They are so young. I think Alex picks up on it the most and he's the one that sees me cry sometimes around Suzanne when I pour my heart out. Well, I have about an hour left and I still need to get the retail race team order ready to fax off tomorrow. I wish I would never run out of words because I seem to be in another world when I'm typing away. I guess because I'm talking to someone even if it's myself.

January 23, 1998. *"Be at peace with yourself"* — I am watching 20/20 about a woman dying of breast Cancer and putting things in order (papers). She wrote a book - a checklist about dying and living. She made videotapes for her young daughter. I was impressed with her courage and faith in God. The fear is not of death but of leaving the love of her husband and child. I'm impressed that everyday is a gift and that death is something that should not be feared. Craig spent the day with Suzanne again. He wanted to walk home and lay down for a while. There were four boxes of crackers out with crackers all over the cupboards, some on the floor and chewed gum on the table and little "wads" of toilet paper in the hallway and bathroom. I put a new roll on this morning and he used the whole roll today. He isn't even home very much. He tried to wash his hands before he ate dinner and flooded the kitchen cupboard and spilled water all over the floor. He just doesn't quite know what to do. He's very possessive and he's consumed with the Clinton news about him having an affair. Steve and Madison called from California. They are at Disneyland. Craig can't quite understand how he can be at Disneyland and talk to us here. All of his reasoning seems to have gone except he remembers he should ice his calves and certain exercises people have told him to do.

January 24, 1998. *"Love always"* — I'm struggling today. Craig is so repetitive and he continues to tell me that Heavenly Father doesn't like me when I lie - that is when I tell him that I know what he's talking about when I don't. So, now I just say I don't know and I believe that flusters him even more. I took him with me this morning to the bank and to open the store. He wanted to talk with Terry for a while. Most of his friends find it hard to carry on an extended conversation. I struggle myself and remind myself that I need to care for me as the caregiver as well. I need to try to stay calm, cool and collected. He breathes almost like he's hyperventilating and says he's sick and all he does is "feces" and that would make anyone sick. I almost think he frightens Alex and Emily at times. Or, at least they don't know what to think at times. Alex, who is 6, said he didn't want to play cards with Grandpa because he doesn't know how. Suzanne just told him Grandpa is sick and he should play with him and help him. Craig flushes the toilet constantly. He just holds the handle down and flushes. I don't know what he thinks he sees but he just watches and watches and flushes and flushes. It's the quiet that is nice once in a while more than the being alone because I feel alone most all of the time anymore. There was a woman that came into the store tonight and was telling me about her neighbor who is 50 and has Alzheimer's and has been in a resthome for the past three years because of his violent behavior. I'm extremely grateful that Craig only gets upset and agitated never angry or violent.

January 25-26, 1998. *"Remember how special you are"* — Yesterday rolled into today. We got up very early yesterday for Craig to go run and for the second Sunday in a row I woke up with a terrible headache and had a hard time getting up and going. I finally got myself together and got dressed for church and then just waited for Craig. He got home around 9:00 and I got him something to eat, shaved and showered him and got him dressed and we went to church. Church is hard too because I never know when he is going to hyperventilate and say he's sick or needs to go to the bathroom. We did make it through and we came home, ate and he laid in the bedroom and watched golf and football until Mel stopped by and I made them some hot chocolate and roll and they watched the last ten minutes of a game while they visited. Craig got upset before we went to bed again when I told him he didn't need to use the bathroom again. I laid awake thinking and finally got up and took a sleeping pill and slept most of the night. I always thought I would live and die in this house with Craig and now the reality of it all is setting in. I've learned the importance of one level as you grow older and I don't feel older. We have one stair from our family room to kitchen. He could not navigate the one stair and would tell me that I was going to feel really bad one day when someone died because of that stair. I want to stay strong but somedays I feel weak and the days are overwhelming.

January 27, 1998. *"Worry does not empty the day of its troubles, but only of its strength"* — Today has been a hard day. Today I took back a little bit of my life. I felt ready for a nervous breakdown after listening to the toilet flush a minimum of 25-30 times from 6 am. to 7 a.m. I got dressed, took half-day vacation and spent the day alone - thinking. I called Giles because he called and talked to Craig last night. I just cried and told him that I was ready to put Craig into a care facility that I just couldn't do it anymore. This morning I did "snap" back at Craig and he was a lot nicer when I brought lunch to him and then made dinner tonight. Debbie's husband picked him up to run at the track tonight. The runners have been so wonderful to pick him up. They only ran five miles and probably slow. I think I'll get him in a hot tub and give him an extra sleeping pill tonight. I have cried so much today and tonight that I'm sure I'll really sleep tonight. Su called Craig tonight and talked to him for probably 30 minutes for a diversion. I visited with Alex. He came over to watch cartoons for 30 minutes and have a cookie and soda. It definitely made me smile and feel good inside. I feel a little rejuvenated tonight. I need to start prioritizing my life and not just Craig's.

January 28, 1998. *"Lighten the load of others"* — This morning I thought would be better. The night was somewhat better, but I gave him two sleeping pills last night and I gave him two tonight. Since he's becoming so agitated I don't quite know what is coming anymore, so at least this allows him to sleep. He didn't like it when I shaved him with the electric razor this morning and wanted me to use the other kind. I told him I needed to buy some more razors. I've decided that even though the electric razor doesn't shave as well it's easier. And, once again I've decided to take some of my own life back or I wouldn't make it to graduation day. Craig told me he hated me and that he doesn't have Alzheimer's and I didn't need to help him do anything and if I hadn't taken his car away he wouldn't need me. Tonight his butt hurt and he wanted some hemorrhoid creams and couldn't quite do it. I reminded him that he didn't want me to help, that he could do things himself. I told him I'd be glad to help if he would ask and be nice. He asked me to help him and then said thanks and walked into the other room. He is concerned about Jamison tonight. They put him into the hospital today with Pneumonia and Craig was very concerned. I had a good talk with Jesse today and told him the extent of how Craig is away from his friends. I also had a good talk with his mother and his sister. Su, who takes care of her mother with Parkinson's disease, has been a big morale booster to me. My friend, Kaylene, called me last night out of the blue and I cried my eyes out. I made a promise to myself to go out once a month and be a friend again. I haven't been a friend or anything else. I have allowed myself to be a prisoner. I need to step back and take control. I've become a different person in the last month. I hope that others can learn from my experiences and that I will be able to help others one day. I intend to call nursing homes and resthomes tomorrow and get price quotes. I would want him to do the same for me. After I tackle tomorrow then I will address the store and taxes. One day at a time, the same as Craig, except I've told Suzanne I need to do that half-day at a time or hour by hour any more. I actually worked at the store this afternoon so Stephen could go to the hospital with Suzanne. Karen, or Carol, as Craig calls her, took him for a run this afternoon and I guess he had a little accident on the trail. She couldn't tell me all of the details because Craig was right there, but it must have been a mess for her and her husband to have to help him clean himself up. She's been great to help with Craig.

January 29, 1998. *"Behave like a duck-calm and unruffled on the surface, but paddle like the devil underneath"* — It was a day of Craig being in better humor, or I should say not so upset. I had him stay home by himself and Jesse picked him up for lunch and then I came home at 3:30. I got a sandwich for him and have started to give him a sleeping pill (Seconol/100Mg) with his anti-depressant at dinner time and a second sleeping pill at around 7:30-8:00. When I got home today his clothes and shoes were everywhere. He said he had to get another roll of toilet paper by himself and he was a little upset. I can't believe he can go through more than one roll a day but he does. I bought him a package of gum tonight so I don't know where his gum is going to end up, but he loves to chew gum. Maybe it takes him back to his baseball days - I hadn't thought of that. He had a conversation with Su again tonight. She's great to let him talk to her for 20 minutes about old school buddies. He told me had something for me and when I asked what it was, he said sex. I told him that was great but I didn't want it. He said he wished I had told him that before we were married. I wanted to laugh, but I couldn't. I did check into "homes" today. There is one in Orem, The Alzheimer's Center. I'm going to check it out next week. I liked the woman that I talked to and it was affordable and it's only Alzheimer residents. I didn't realize that a lot of "homes" would not take Alzheimer's patients. They say that it is because they wander and get violent, but I've decided it's because they can't get Medicare and Medicaid for them. It is truly a wicked disease. I hope that by writing this so-called diary that it will help someone else with the day-to-day questions of some other young (relatively speaking) Alzheimer's caregiver. I feel stronger today and feel at peace in knowing that there is a place with a wonderful caring environment for Craig to live. Now, we'll face that bridge when we come to it. I've been a caregiver and not much of anything else these past years. When people ask me about myself, I remind them that I have a lifetime for me and this time belongs to Craig. Little by little we are all coming together with our thoughts. I knew we would. We've always been supportive of each other. I'm excited to spend an evening with Suzanne and Wendy. I'm going to get bolder and stronger. I told Steve I'm keeping a diary and documenting his dad's disease. I want to entitle it " The Diary of a Young Caregiver" — that may change as I seek help from someone as I finish it. My hope is that I can help someone understand the days and how they differ with all the little weird things they do as the disease progresses. I don't want to forget all of the crazy little things he's done and does. I found out about an article in a magazine that someone wrote about him and "Big Al" — tomorrow I probably won't write, but Saturday should be interesting after spending an evening out both for Craig with Steve and the girls and myself out for an evening with the Alzheimer's Association. I'm looking forward to meeting people that I have talked to over the past two years.

January 30-31, 1998. *"Ulcers aren't what you eat, it's what's eating you"* — Friday was a great day. Not only did I dress in a suit and it felt good, but I spent the night with my two daughters, Suzanne and Wendy. We went to an Alzheimer's black-tie fundraiser. It was a wonderful night just spending time with them. We sat at the head table with the master of ceremonies and one of the doctors of gerontology who was honored. It was interesting to get different views of people. He said the most important aspect of a support group is that you get various viewpoints for different aspects of the disease. I know I want to hear about people's view on care facilities and other coping mechanisms. Today I worked at the store and visited with Richard. He just put his mother in a care facility today with Alzheimer's. After talking with him I know that when that day comes it is going to have to be a friend who takes him and not me or one of the children. He said his mother just shouted obscenities at them and told them she hated them. To know that I was leaving Craig somewhere to live and not ever bringing him home and hear those things, I don't know if I could handle it. I know that day is fast approaching. So many aspects of my life will change as I contemplate selling the store and starting life in new surroundings by myself. The doctor last night said that if I never publish the diary I am writing or the documentation that I am doing each night is that it is very therapeutic for me. I feel like I'm talking from my heart each day to someone. I've decided that I need to take a portion of my life back. I need to keep sane. I need time away and I need to seek out and ask for help more often. As a Caregiver I know that I need to care for myself physically and emotionally. And, when you consider there are an estimated four million Americans that have this degenerative disease that affects their ability to functional normally and to remember who they are and the people and places they've known for decades, there are a lot of us, Caregivers, out there. We went to a dinner for Manu's son tonight. Craig enjoys being around him and his friends and family. They dearly love Craig.

In talking to Richard today he said he doesn't even know Craig anymore. The Craig he knows would never swear or say an unkind thing. Now we never know what is coming out of his mouth. I told him that I have never been afraid of Craig being abusive. He gets upset and angry from time to time, but I think he is angrier with himself because he can't do things for himself. I told him not to worry because it only had to happen once and I've checked into facilities. I found a wonderful place (I think). I drove by there and I really liked the woman on the phone and the literature she sent. I need to visit this next week. Well I'm hoping that after not sleeping last night, I will be able to sleep better tonight.

Suzanne surprised me by saying that she wanted to speak at her Dad's funeral and Wendy said Steve wants to and I told her that we should because we are all his best friends and Wendy and Stephen could say prayers. It was a neat feeling knowing that they want to share in the final testament of love.

February 1, 1998. *"Smile and the world smiles back."* — Today was a hard day. I thought I was going to have a nervous breakdown. Craig thought there was feces in his cereal and feces on the floor. He used a dozen paper towels to take it out of his cereal. It was bite size shredded wheat and had brown specks. I hadn't mopped the floor and whatever he saw on the floor was feces. Then he had to use the bathroom every five minutes. His friends, Bob and Richard, picked him up to run and just getting him ready was a nightmare. I was so tired from the night before that I took a sleeping pill and slept off and on and got up at 6:15 to get him ready. Their run was shorter this morning. I'm sure it's harder each week for them to run and then take him to have juice. I hadn't had time to get in the tub before he got back. I got ready to go to church and then called Mike and asked him to pick Craig up and take him. I ended up not going. I stayed home, got in the tub, and just sat on the couch in the quiet and read a little. I've got so I don't even like the noise of the television. I've got to talk to the children this week after I visit this facility and tell them that I'm ready to have a nervous breakdown and I don't know how much longer I can do this. I am going to go to the support group this Wednesday. Perhaps they will help with some of the questions I have about care facilities. I'm reading "An Alzheimer's Anthology" that I got at the fundraiser the other night — interesting.

February 2-3, 1998. *"The size of our troubles depend on if they are coming or going"* — Monday was a hard day with Craig wanting his butt wiped every ten minutes and four pairs of dirty underwear when I got home and soda spilled everywhere and having him tell me how much he dislikes everything. I told him it was hard for me too, and I think it must have got to him because when Karen brought him back from running and having dinner with her and her family he apologized and said he would be nice. This morning he told me just to let him know when to get up for breakfast. Usually, he demands he needs food. My doctor friend told me he would get me some names of someone that could come in and help care for Craig in the mornings. It would eliminate some stress. Bob and Richard are picking him up for lunch today. They are thoughtful. They take him to the same place each week and order the same food. I'm going to go to the show with Steve and Wendy at 4:00 and see the movie Titanic. I had dinner last night with Wendy and the girls. It was fun.

We went to the Tepanyaki restaurant and had a great time. Craig has had a better day with me here. I still don't know what he does with his underwear. He must just take them off and drop them in the tub. I know he doesn't know how to turn the water in the tub to rinse them out and they are always just in a wet heap on the floor. He always thinks he stinks and wants to wash his hands. He washes them but never dries them. I need to get some of the new soapless soap that doesn't need to be rinsed off. It is definitely like a little child. You devise methods to avoid certain behaviors. He's very picky about the shoes he wears to run. When I was getting him ready to go to the track he said he needed his racing flats on. He also says he stinks which means he wants me to put deodorant on for him. It was good to stay home today. I feel calmer and almost inspired as to what I need to do. I've cried until I can't cry any more. I came home to meet Craig and dirty towels all over. I got him in the tub, washed his hair and told him to soak. I gave him two sleeping pills and I hope he sleeps. He's not only repetitive but has continual questions. Much like a little child that keeps repeating "what's that?" He thinks I'm the person to fill in for everyone and that I need to tell people I can't do it. I don't know where that came from.

February 4, 1998. *"Catch the vision"* — Today I didn't work and stayed home but at noon worked at the store so Stephen and Suzanne could be with Stephen's brother as he got ready to depart for his mission. Brett is wonderful and is always there to help me. He came in at 2:00 and stayed until 4:00 when Patrick came in. Pat and Vaughn are two "wonders" that never cease to amaze me. That freed me up to go home to Craig. Craig had a couple of accidents while I was gone. I think I'm getting used to cleaning up "feces" after him. He tries to clean up himself but it just makes it worse. He apologizes but he just doesn't understand. This morning I had to give him an extra anti-depressant because I couldn't get him to quit crying. He said he was so stupid that he wanted to kill himself. It took quite a while this morning to settle him down. I ran a pizza home to him and he said it was the best food he's had. It must have tasted good to him for a change. Craig had dinner with Suzanne and the children tonight while I went to dinner with a friend. You never imagine that you are going to have your children or anyone for that matter tend your spouse while you go out with a friend.

February 5, 1998. *"Have the courage of your desire"* — I'm sitting here with Craig watching television, his favorite: Larry King – Larry King Live he says. He is interviewing a reverend. He said that indeed good things do happen to good people and it is with the love of the Lord that they are strengthened and have joy and peace with all their trials. I do find peace with the love and help from my children and Craig's wonderful friends. We called Su tonight. Craig said he couldn't remember who she is because all he did was play baseball and he thinks she was one of the "wild" ones. We sat by her at our last class reunion, but he doesn't remember. He is so consumed with his sore bum all the time and I don't know what he's done today with himself but his underwear is on backwards and I know that I put it on him this morning right. The nightstand was pulled away from the wall and I don't know what he does with things when he is here by himself. Darkness frightens him. He can't find his way at all in the dark. You have to leave a light on at night so he can see if he wakes up. He gets anxious when I type away at night. I told him it's because I can't go to work as early in the morning so I need to do this at night. He said that's crap and when I reminded him that I need to help him in the morning he didn't believe me. He said I could put him on a train instead. I asked him where he wanted me to send him when he was on the train and he said heaven. I just want to be swept away myself. Calgon take me away. Actually, I wish someone would take Craig away for a day and let me just have a day alone to come and go and have the house to myself with no sounds, no questions, no nothing. I know that I say these things and that one-day, all too soon, I will be by myself, and there will be days when I'll wish I could listen to him and care for him. Tonight he is just rattling on and on. He wants to know what every mark on his leg or anything anywhere is and why. He thinks he's had surgery everywhere and he hates himself. I have no idea what he is talking about half the time anymore. I've got to see about getting help in the mornings with him and let someone else shave, shower and dress him and let me be able to just walk away some mornings. Trials are what make us strong and believers in Christ and Christlike as we endeavor to move forward. I thought I believed I was strong and had learned a lot already. I hope the rest of my life will be with fewer trials, or not big ones anyway — only little ones. I want my life to be simple and take care of Craig. I don't want to live to be 108 but I do hope the second half of my life is as fulfilling as the first. I don't know if I could handle being a caregiver another time.

February 6, 1998. *"If the eyes didn't have tears the heart wouldn't have rainbows"* — The end of the week. I don't know where the week went but it's gone. I've enjoyed working for Jack. At least I know I have a job right now. I went to visit The Alzheimer's Center, a facility in Orem today. I really liked the woman that is over the center and they eat family style, have a large fenced yard with a picnic table, and they have people in to dance or work out with the patients. It takes up to twenty people and all with Alzheimer's. I've decided that like Suzanne, we need to wait until Craig no longer knows us. I almost pray for that day to come and yet when it does I don't know what I'll do. He was so loving and cute with Jamison tonight. He loves the children and is so happy that Emily is better. Wendy and Madison brought him lunch today and he remembered who brought lunch and said he thought that was very nice of them to do that. I've decided for the time being it's easier to have him stay home and have someone check on him than taking him somewhere every day. He knows the routine of our house and he knows where the bathroom is. I think that is a comfort to him. I have started to double the anti-depressants in the morning and at dinner time I give him another one with a sleeping pill around 7:00-8:00. He's aware that tomorrow he is going to go run with the team. It is such a hassle, but worth it, I guess. I know it is hard on whoever is the one dedicated to run with him. I've got to figure out what to do with the store. I'm hoping that if I do the things that I am supposed to do each day and remain Christlike that the Lord will bless me and help me make it through each day. I pray for strength...God help me know what to do. I pray for a miracle not knowing what a miracle even is anymore.

February 7, 1998. *"Nothing we wear makes as much difference as our facial expression"* — I've decided that as much as I have always loved being busy and have a lot going on, I am looking forward to emptying my plate and being my own person. I did get my tax information assembled tonight and balanced my checkbook and wrote out bills. I feel like I got everything done tonight that I was going to do tomorrow. I really want to go to church with Wendy and the girls tomorrow and so I knew I needed to get this done tonight. I am going to send Craig to Stake Conference with the neighbors and stay home. He went running this morning with the race team for about eight miles and then came back for muffins and juice and visiting. I then took him home to shower and dress and took him up to his mother's to visit. Patty brought him home at 5:30 and I closed the store at 6:00 and came home and fixed him dinner. We called Su and he chatted for 20 minutes. She calls and talks to Craig so that I can go get in the tub for an undisturbed 15-minute bubble bath. It's heaven. She's been an angel. I'm excited for her to speak before the legislature on the 11th on the aging. I think he was tired from the run and getting up early so I gave him sleeping meds early and it's 10:00 and he's been out for a good hour. I'm sure that tomorrow morning will come all too soon when we get up early to get him ready to run.

February 8, 1998. *"You can't make a second first impression"* — I let Craig sleep in today and not go run with his friends. He slept all through the night. I think his long run and two sleeping pills helped. It was nice. I called and told Bob and Richard not to pick him up. I told him they called and decided not to run. He got up at 8:30 in time to not rush, eat and get ready to go to conference with the neighbors. It was nice to have two hours alone. I never know what I do anymore other than the fact that the day comes and goes. I wanted to go to church with Wendy and the girls, but they must have forgotten and gone somewhere. They weren't home. I stopped by the store and just sat there for 30 minutes in the quiet and now here I am by myself typing away. I'd read but I just am not able to concentrate. Bill called tonight again to talk to him. He amazes me with his kindness to Craig. He calls at least once a week and just chatters away with him. He and Doris are always kind to call and invite us to go eat with them on Sundays for a little outing as well. I wish I could take a pill and sleep for a week or maybe a month. Actually, I would just like to run away for maybe a day.

February 9, 1998. *"There is always tomorrow"* — Today was a day of reckoning with myself (mostly). Suzanne helps me see things and put things into perspective. I've really been struggling lately. She said, "Mom,

I don't know what we need to do, but we can't put dad in a home yet. He still knows everyone." I told her I know that and I agree, but I just feel overwhelmed lately. On some days I wished I could just stay home and take care of him every day; but I also feel like I need to maintain a life in order to help myself and thus help Craig. We decided that it's too early to put Craig into a home and that it's best to keep him at home and have someone check on him and bring him in lunch.

February 10, 1998. *"Contentment consists of few wants"* — I'm sitting alone. Craig isn't back from running. Debbie, Karen and Jeannie from the race team picked him up and took him to the track and over to Paul's for a rubdown. Suzanne was feeling down tonight and I told her at least we take turns having our down days. I wish I had a bunch of money and oh what fun I could have doing for others. I think that would be the best part of having money. I took half day off this afternoon and came home to be with Craig and fix him a sandwich before he went to run. Jesse picked him up and took him to lunch today. So, I ate lunch alone while I watched the news. I pray for strength each day. Craig amazes me with some of his statements. Today when he got up he said he woke up in the night and talked to Heavenly Father and told him to make Alex well because he is such a fine/good boy. Alex was sick the day before. Then he talked about Jamison and how happy he makes him because he smiles at him. It's amazing the little things as a child's smile that so thrills you.

February 12, 1998. *"If you can think of nothing for which to give thanks, you have a poor memory"* — It's been a good day. Work is still strained while going through a merger. We listened to Larry King, whose guest went through drug and alcohol abuse treatment and lost a child. He said that he "wore" his friends out talking about his grief. I thought that was a great choice of words—wore my friends out—before I sought professional help. He went in once a week and talked to someone. I understood completely. I think that is why your friends stay away when you get life-threatening illnesses and something like Alzheimer's. They don't relate and thus they don't know what to say or how to "listen." "Listen" is a key word too. Some of Craig's friends thought I was embellishing how Craig was slipping because he could talk to them for a period of time and "looks" good; but they don't see him for long periods of time and see what I see and hear. I've decided that also, they talk to Craig, but they don't really listen or they would know. It makes you internalize more. Steve calls me at work to talk to me. He still calls his dad at nights but if he wants to really talk to me we do it away from Craig. I wish today were Friday. I've decided the days are easier when I can spend more time at home with Craig.

February 13, 1998. *"If you scatter thorns don't go barefoot"* — The end of the week....sort of. Craig told me this morning that he knew it was my birthday coming up because he saw Emily put it on the calendar. And, Suzanne said we are all going to dinner on Sunday but I may not be able to go because I'm a "butt-hole." I told him that wasn't nice and he said can't you take a joke? He stayed at home most of the day and went back and forth to Suzanne's and went around the block with them. He's talking to Su for his nightly call. It's funny to hear him talk to her about their high school days and say, "I can't believe I don't know who you are or what you look like." He said he wanted to take her to lunch if I would get him a car or give him the keys to mine. I think he's definitely reverting backwards. He constantly says he needs to use the bathroom or asks me if he needs to. I tell him no, that he just went. It's every five minutes he says he needs to go. I try to remind him that he just went. I feel like my life is falling more and more into place with a peace inside that I haven't felt until these past few days. As I wake up in the night, I find myself asking for help from God to sleep. I almost feel like I sound like Craig. He tells me he wakes up in the night and talks to Heavenly Father. Hopefully, God is preparing us both. I know that I have a lot of work to do to fulfill my mission here on this earth. Bonnie called me today to wish me a happy birthday. It's hard to believe that I will be 55 tomorrow. I told Steve I feel like 23 if that counts. I really do feel much younger than I used to think 55 was. This week has been an eye opener week. I'm more at peace with myself, learned the phrase "wore out my friends," and they aren't "listening" when they hear Craig talk if they think he's okay and that I'm embellishing how bad he is. I guess after two years of watching the decline I want people to know how tragic it is and about the disease. So,

I tell people all of the crazy things he says and does hoping that they will understand or at least have some understanding of what it is like to live with him. He truly is close to the other side when you think he has no cares. He's on anti-depressants, stays home all day or with someone taking care of him constantly, dressing, shaving, and feeding. He has no concerns or worries of life. He's just waiting for his Father in Heaven to take him home. I really hope that it isn't a long wait so that he can start preparing for the rest of us and help us all out from the other side. I think Grandpa and Grandma Hanseen are anxiously waiting for their "boy" to join them.

February 14, 1998. *"To err is human, to forgive is divine"* — Well today is my birthday, 55. Alex and Emily came over early and brought me a scrapbook. Steve stopped by and gave me a cute stuffed animal for my toy collection. I then went to work at the store for the morning. Wendy, Taylor and Madison stopped by and brought me another stuffed animal to put with my toys at home. We had a fun visit at the store. Wendy brought her mother with them. I am so blessed that our children married such wonderful people and blessed us with such choice grandchildren. Mike and Linda picked Craig up and then came to the store and got me. We went for a birthday lunch. It was fun and probably more laughs for them than for me. It's hard when you are in public and are trying to care for his needs and have it appear effortless so others don't know. They dropped me off at the store and I worked the rest of the day. Suzanne took Alex to the hospital because of his stomach pain. He has a bowel obstruction. I guess we are still on for tomorrow. Craig rattles more and more. He literally made no sense at all today. He talks about all the shoes he's found and being green when he was sick with Alzheimer's. He said a little prayer tonight for Alex. I know that I need patience with Craig, which I seem to have been blessed with this past two weeks. I don't think much could throw me right now. I say that but I don't really know that. Tonight when I got home Craig had his coat on and said he was cold and his bum was sore and he needed help. As soon as I said Alex was sick then it was like he didn't need or command as much attention. Perhaps I should write this at the end as a "life with Big Al" and concentrate on the humor in it instead of just a day-to-day journal. He seems to have a harder time with the telephone lately. He doesn't quite know what to do with it. We have a "hands free" model in the kitchen and Craig calls it a cellular and he said he tried to call me one morning and I never would talk back. Suzanne asked him if the phone ever rang or did he get a dial tone and he said he didn't know, but that he cussed at me because I never would answer him.

February 25, 1998. *"Smile and change it or grin and bear it"* — Craig spent the day out on his own (wandering). The neighbor called Suzanne about 9:00 (right after I left for work) and told her that her dad was down on her front yard looking lost. He wanted to visit Edna around the corner and he couldn't remember where she lived. She is the mother of an old school mate of ours. I'm surprised she let him in to talk. Yesterday he changed his clothes and went running and actually made it home. I do not know how he ever accomplished this. He literally cannot dress himself and then he came home and showered and put his clothes back on. He said the only thing he couldn't do was this and he pointed to his hair. He didn't know how to brush his hair. I have a feeling this is only the beginning. We've been blessed.

February 26-27, 1998. *"Make happy those who are near"* — Thursday I came home early and went with friends to dinner. It was nice to be away, but I always feel like I am gone too long and never quite relax and enjoy my time away. Bob and Richard picked Craig up yesterday and took him to lunch. They are good friends. They try to take him to the same place and order him the same food each time. Mel stopped by and helped Craig organize his shoes and found one he thought was lost. He had 22 pairs of running shoes all lined up and is so proud of them. If he only knew I've given half of them away to charity this past summer along with a lot of our clothes. I'm trying to sort out as much as I can. He also has a lot of socks and Steve said he has enough. I'm trying to move forward with getting rid of the store. Between the store and the race team it's getting to be too much. My plate is too full and I need to be eliminating things, as Craig needs more of my time and energy. Last night I woke up every hour except for the hour when Craig was in the bathroom. He missed the toilet and hollered for me to help him. I dried him off, changed his clothes, cleaned the bathroom floor and put him back to bed. He looked up and said "thank you for getting up to help me - I love you." He's appreciative when you help him. He's gotten soft and kind again like the "old" Craig. He wanted to go running tonight when I got home. I helped him change his clothes. He came back three times before I thought he was out and gone and here he came back. He made it to the corner and had a little accident. I threw away the pants like the other accidents and had him get in the tub and then eat some dinner. Mike and Linda stopped by to visit and he showed his rows of shoes he was so proud of. Oh, I hope I sleep tonight. I want to go to bed and not wake until morning.

February 28, 1998. *"Love truth"* — The same old Saturday. I worked at the store and Craig stayed home with Suzanne checking on him and bringing him lunch. Manu picked him up and took him to a family party. He didn't have time to take him home so he brought him to the store. He was amazed at all the new shoes and tried to talk to Stephen. I took him home then went back. I had a good talk with Mike and Linda on my way home and Linda thinks he's slipped a lot in the last month. He's consumed about his bowels and bathroom habits and eating — two things he doesn't do well by himself. He just spilled his hot chocolate all down him on his robe. I gave him a blanket and he spilled mine on the blanket. So, now he's gone and got a coat of his and put it on over his underclothes. I want to laugh but I can't.

I don't know if I said this earlier. But one night when I got home late he had his underclothes on backwards and said he couldn't believe these things had holes. So, the next day I put them on backwards and he asked me who had "Big Al," him or me? We're waiting for Su to call back and talk to him after she gets her mother to bed. He wanted to kneel down and say a prayer for her mother. He talks to the Lord rather freely like he's right there beside him, and in a lot of ways, I suppose he is. Suzanne fed the missionaries tonight and brought her dad over a plate of food to eat. She is so sweet with her dad. I've always loved Norman Rockwell and I used to love to put puzzles together. She brought me a Norman Rockwell puzzle today to put together. It made me feel all good inside. She is such a blessing in my life.

March 7, 1998. *"A gem cannot be polished without friction"* — Steve just called. He sounds wonderful. He seems more relaxed. He has so much to give and has such a big heart. I would love it if he could find the same peace that I have. Life is funny how it plays out. We have always been hard workers — every one of us.

The other night we had a neighbor stop by and Craig went on to explain that when he was first diagnosed and took all the "tests" that he didn't even know what year it was or how old he was. Now he knows all that stuff. I asked him what year it was and he said 39. I said 39 what? 1939? And he said yes isn't that right and I told him it was and our neighbor just winked and smiled. I asked him how old he was and said forty and that he's getting right up there but at least he's not as old as I am. I'm 55 and I told him I was 53 and he didn't say anything.

March 8, 1998. *"Everyone is a house with four rooms, a physical, a mental, an emotional and a spiritual. Most of us tend to live in one room most of the time, but unless we go into every room every day, even if only to keep it aired, we are not a complete person."* – An Indian Proverb — He wanted me to sit out his running clothes and I told him I would come home for lunch and help him. He dressed by himself. He stopped by to tell Suzanne and he had three shirts on and she helped him take one off. We knew he had his necklace on and that the weather was pretty nice. He was gone for about two hours and said he ran into some lady and told her he had Alzheimer's and did she know where he lived because he was a little mixed up. I don't know who she was but she guided him home. Someone from the neighborhood called Suzanne and said that he was up in the tree streets and out in the middle of the road. My biggest fear is that someone will hit him when he's out by himself.

He did run with the race team yesterday. Terry said what they need for the races this summer is something on his shirt that says, "guide runner" and then have he and Craig attached somehow by their arms. Craig gets very confused in crowds and he could get lost very easy. Craig is becoming looser in his speech with people — just talking to anyone and everyone. I have to tell him not to talk so loud. Friday he told me that he hated this disease and that he wanted to go live with Heavenly Father. I told him it wasn't that easy and that we would all like to go live with Heavenly Father.

March 9, 1998. *"Something good will be found in this day"* — Craig has had a fun day with our friend, Mark. He is travelling through with his daughter, Tawney, to Los Angeles. He is so good with Craig and to Craig. It makes my heart feel so good and it also makes my heart cry because I remember the friendship they had when Craig was Craig, before Big Al took over. I think of him as a sick child that I worry about when he is away or I'm away. I know that he is enjoying himself with Mark. I'm waiting for them to come back home. Craig will talk about it for days—possibly weeks. You never know any more. They came to visit me at work and Craig remembered people. One of my friends hugged me and cried and couldn't say anything. She hadn't seen Craig since he got sick. Craig just seems to decline but yet he still seems to know each of us. He just can't do things as simple as sitting on the couch or sitting on the chair to eat at the table. I wish at times he could go tomorrow and at times I love just knowing that he is here even though he's not here. I know that he loves me and I have learned so much from him since this illness. The Lord definitely works in strange ways. I definitely know that most of Craig's work will be done on the other side. I also know how nice it is to have an hour of quiet by myself. I never realized the extent until I have that time by myself. Craig's memory of things never ceases to amaze me as well. He remembers things but won't be able to associate a name with which he is talking about and so he'll attempt to describe them in some way until you finally know what he is talking about. Mark talked about his experience of taking Craig to a public restroom today. He experienced how he starts to undress before he even gets to the restroom. Also, he doesn't stand to urinate, but Mark somehow got him to do that today. I'm sure he's had some laughs as well as tears today. I'd love to know what is going on in Craig's mind, if he has glimpses of normalcy or not.

It's midnight and I just got Craig into bed. I gave him two sleeping pills and he sat in the hot tub at Steve and Wendy's with Mark and then he has been with Mark and Tawney all day. I'm sure he's very tired because he was hallucinating when he got into the bed. Tawney said he had his shoes on the wrong feet when they stopped by to pick him up. I cried my heart out when they left. It's so nice to have people around that love him and then when they leave I feel like I'm in life alone again. I don't quite know what to do anymore — one day at a time. I don't know what a life is but I'm not sure that when I get one that I will miss the taking care of Craig as I know it today.

March 10, 1998. *"Each day is a gift to be treasured"* — Su, our little angel, is talking to Craig. Debbie and Ron picked him up and took him to the track to run. He came home, ate and got in the tub with his sleeping medication and is now doing his little nightly chat with Su. Suzanne said he wanted to go running today but she told him he couldn't that it was too cold. I'm dreading the summer already. He is determined to run and he doesn't even know how to dress himself. As he talked to Bill at night he said he's ready to play golf every day too. I have so many feelings inside me right now. I feel blessed and overwhelmed all at the same time. I guess I need to learn to live each day with a prayer in my heart.

March 11, 1998. *"Great opportunities come to those who make the most of small ones"* — Craig went to visit his mother today for a few hours. He had lunch with Suzanne and spent most of the day at home. I came home early and took him to get his hair washed and trimmed. It always makes him feel good. Camille is sweet to do that for Craig. We came home, ate dinner and Craig hurried because he wanted to visit with Kelsch while I went to the store. But, he closed early and so Craig had to go to the store with me. That is not a pleasant task. He likes to push the cart and doesn't know where he is going. Then he likes to help load and unload and that's even worse. The last time he tried to help put them in the car and the bag-boy was there helping. He just looked at me with a blank look when Craig didn't know how to pick the sacks up and when he did he would drop them and the groceries would roll down the parking lot. There is nothing you can say in front of him excep, "That's okay, we drop them too." When we got home I went into Suzanne's and visited with Craig and let her unload the groceries away from Craig so he wouldn't want to help. It's amazing the little things we take for granted. I need to call the church paper and have them put a little blurb in the ward news about Craig wandering now that the weather is such that he will want to run more. Craig is still obsessed each day with his sore bum and going to the bathroom.

March 12, 1998. *"As we have therefore opportunity, let us do good unto all men…"* (Galatians 5:10) - Craig went out running today and Suzanne didn't know. She called me and said she thought he had been gone for a couple of hours then. I went home at noon and Emily was outside and said, "Judy, we already found Grandpa Craig and he is walking with a friend and then he'll be home." I went and "rounded" him up. She said they had walked for three hours and he had passed her twice before she recognized him. She said he took some stairs and the road pretty good. He wants to get up early tomorrow to run so that he doesn't link up with any "walkers" because he needs to run. I think I'll try to go to work late tomorrow. The children hugged our necks and said we were the best grandma and grandpa ever. Craig talked to himself the whole time he was in the tub tonight. He said he was practicing for what he was going to tell Su when she calls. When I helped him get dressed he said to put the pants on right so his "tinkle" would be right. He's coming up with some words lately that are so funny. Sometimes it's all I can do to keep a straight face.

March 14, 1998. *"Look for ways to serve others"* — Another Saturday. Craig went out running and said he was gone for three and a half-hours. I don't know for sure since we don't know when he left or came home. He said he knows every route and doesn't get lost. He now wants a scale to see if he's fat. He doesn't know its called a scale - just that its something that tells you if you're fat and we could get one from the old person's store and not pay very much. He gets obsessed with some of the funniest things. He is so proud when he comes home and he feels like he's accomplished something by himself. He just grins and it makes you feel good. It's been a busy day dealing with insurance adjusters most of the day and then retelling the story. People have been unbelievably good about it. We had a pretty good day considering. I came home and ate lunch with Craig and I saw Carl this morning and had a nice visit with him. He is a very good person. I know everyone has his or her challenges each day. Today Craig got himself dressed alone and was so proud but he didn't have his underclothes on. He said he knew something was different but he couldn't figure it out. He doesn't know how to put his bottoms on the right way. Right now he's missing his gum. I can't find it anywhere. I can't think that he would have chewed a whole giant package.

March 15, 1998. *"The only thing that comes without effort is age"* — Craig and I watched the movie, Slingblade. It made me cry as I thought of someone with a low mentality with such a big heart and so moral knowing right from wrong. It reminded me of how Craig is now. I cried a lot. I feel like I need to protect Craig and I want to be so patient and kind as I spend these last days with him.

Craig is going to day care tomorrow at The Alzheimer's Center. I'm nervous that he won't like it like the last one. Except this time he's a little more advanced into the disease and we've talked a lot more about 'volunteering' than before. There is a gentleman around 63 that can carry on a conversation like Craig can, but he can't use a toothbrush. It pretty much describes Craig. He was talking about his surgery he had, Colonoscopy, and he said when he had his tinkle done was he all right? It is definitely like Charades when you talk to him. Mike picked him up and took him to church. I wanted him to be late so that they could announce about Craig out and about running by himself during the day. I'm not nervous about him getting lost for some reason. For most of everything anymore I have a peace about me. I pray that tomorrow goes well. I am going to take half day off on Tuesday and Wednesday and try to get caught up with things. I need to get my snow tires off and I don't have time to get anything done. Craig was so thrilled when he came home from running yesterday and he got himself undressed and dressed. The only thing was that he didn't have his underclothes on. He said, "Oh, I knew something was missing but I couldn't figure out what." Today he went running with his friends and came home and talked about his sore butt again. I know one day I'm going to be lost.

March 16, 1998. *"Kindness is always becoming"* — Today was a day when Craig spent half-day 'volunteering' at The Alzheimer's Center. He was a little nervous, but was anxious to "help." He told me if I didn't pick him up on time it would be like "Slingblade" — a movie we watched last night about a guy that chopped two people's heads and they locked him in an institution then released him. He read the bible and knew what was right and wrong and had a kind heart. I went for a ride just to cry after I watched the movie. It made me even more protective of Craig. He's so fragile and so in need of someone to help him all the time. I told him that if he were thinking of "slingblading" me he would have to live at The Alzehimer's Center because there wouldn't be anyone at home to take care of him. He told me "just kidding." He thinks he was there helping others out. They liked him and he liked them. He said he doesn't want to go back anytime too soon; but he wouldn't mind going once in a while to help. He told me I had to take my turn 'volunteering' too. I asked him if he would like it better if we got paid for it and thought I could give him $5 each time he went. He said he's sure that Heavenly Father liked it that he was helping people. He said he felt sorry for them and how lucky he is that he has these two little white pills. He said they had him "tinkle" while someone watched and then something about a card. I couldn't figure that one out. The tinkle part was they probably had him urinate standing and anymore it's easier and less accidents if I have him pull his pants down and sit. It is getting harder for him to understand how to pull his pants up though. He said he helped one guy rub his shin splits out and then said another guy knew his uncle, Pratt. One guy told him he was handsome. He got embarrassed and I told him it was true. He said he didn't think so with his "shit hair". He told him that Heavenly Father would help them and that we were raising money for Alzheimer's and wanted to make them feel good. He said the one guy needed help with his "whiner" — Craig said, "What do you think he means by that— I don't know what a whiner is?" I told him I didn't know and I could hardly control laughing. I didn't let him see me smile. When Steve called to check on him he told him all about his day of volunteering and the guy with the 'whiner' problem and did he know what it was he was talking about. Steve told him and then Craig told me I was sure dumb. (I assured Steve I knew what he was talking about and just trying to go to another subject). Then one lady really got mad when they didn't feed her. He said he was on his feet all day long helping people and one guy wanted to know if he could drive. He told him he couldn't that he had Alzheimer's too. He came home feeling pretty lucky. I picked him up at 3:00 and brought him home and let him go run for a while. He came home an hour later and had a little accident. He said not too bad, it's just one little ball and he wanted to drop it out for someone. I told him that wasn't nice. He actually passed Alex coming home through the park from school but he didn't know who he was. Craig was nervous, I'm sure, with a little cluster of children and ran on the grass. Strange as it seems, I think he found his way home by himself today. He keeps telling me that his head is blowing up. He said it was quite a day of talking a lot and asking everyone how they were doing and he felt really good about it. He thinks that's why he has a headache. And, he keeps telling me about this guy's "whiner." I can't wait for him to talk to Su tonight and listen to what he has to tell her. Now, he's saying maybe it hurts because of the Tylenol or it's the Tylenol that hurts. There is a little kid crying on the television on a commercial and he said "that's how I feel buddy" — he talks to himself a lot lately and rattles even more. When he has gas he just starts hollering "mercy" — I don't think he knows the difference between gas and a feeling of a real bowel movement any more. I think that's why he has his little accidents while he is out running.

March 17, 1998. *"There is no right way to do the wrong thing"* — We just got back from his sister's home. It was her birthday. We had a nice visit. Craig went to lunch with Jesse today and then I came home and helped him change his clothes so he could run for a little bit. I took half day off to play catch-up. I've got a doctor appointment tomorrow with my oncologist and I'm a little nervous. I don't know what I would do if the Big C came back before Craig graduates. Craig was anxious to share his story about The Alzheimer's Center.

March 18, 1998. *"Make sunshine all year"* — Stephen had food poisoning or the flu and Patrick and Klint both had school; so, I was the store employee today. I went to work, took care of voice mail, email and faxes, etc. then went to the store. We had a whopping $200 day. (We had a fire at the store and I've been so pre-occupied with my days with Craig that I've never mentioned it). I was up one morning early when Steve called at 6:00 and said to turn the television on, that our store was on fire. I called Stephen and Suzanne and she said Stephen had been there all night when he got the call at midnight. Craig was a good friend with most of the firefighters and they knew Stephen was running the store and called him. They knew there was no sense in calling me because I couldn't leave Craig alone at night. It's frightening for the days ahead of remodeling for a two to three week period. It will be interesting to see how the insurance works out and how long it takes to get paid for the remodeling. We definitely need to get rid of the smoke smell. Craig went running by himself today and once again made it back. Suzanne turned the water on for him and set his clothes out for him, fed him lunch and then some soup and told him I would be home with pizza for dinner. He's anxious and nervous about going to the care center again to help. He said he has a life too and he needs to help with Alex and Emily and mostly Jamison. I try to be as patient as I can but he thinks I get upset with him. I did get him in the tub to soak and cut his hair a little bit. He's talking to Su and she's going to try to talk him into going to daycare tomorrow. I told him that maybe they would pay him to help and he didn't like that idea either. He said he has a life and that I need to take a turn volunteering more. I got a clean bill of health today when I went in for my Cancer checkup.

March 19, 1998. *"I will give myself the gift of personal time today"* — Craig went to day care again today. I picked him up at 3:45 and he was in the dining room talking to two other residents. He was telling them that they needed to take Vitamin E, that it helps the most. He said that Pratt (the fellow that said he knew his uncle) was really mean today. He told him to shut-up. Craig didn't like that. He said he doesn't want to go back any time soon because those people aren't very smart or they would be giving them Vitamin E, because that's what people with Alzheimer's are supposed to have. He said the people that help are just too young and not smart enough. He tried to help the one guy on with his sweater at the end of the day and then he said, "Oh, let my wife help you instead because she helps me and she's faster than I am even though I could probably do it." They sent him home with some frosted animal cookies (baggie) for his grandchildren. Craig said that one woman kept asking him if he was going to hurt her and he kept asking, "why would I want to hurt you." Craig doesn't realize how often he asks the same thing. I kept laughing when he was telling me about his day. Actually he was laughing as well. He came home and went running and found his way home again. He wasn't gone very long and had another little accident. He said it wasn't bad because it was strong. He said he thought about stopping in the gutter. I told him never to do that because it isn't nice. Oh, I can only imagine. He said he likes to run by himself when he isn't tired because he knows his own routes the best.

He is still wondering why Steve one night told him to be nice to Mom. Craig was confused. I believe that by finding peace within myself I've had a sense of peace about assisting Craig and feeling the honor that it is to serve him. As he becomes more child-like he is like a kid in that he senses who loves him and who doesn't. I think that's why he is so into Jamison because Jamison just beams because he knows his Grandpa loves him and Craig knows that he loves him.

March 21, 1998. *"Have a song in your heart"* — Yesterday I actually went out after work and went to a movie with Sue. I felt guilty leaving Craig alone for so long. I have such mixed feelings as to having a life of my own and being here to be with Craig when he needs me, or maybe it's just may be that I feel more needed — interesting thought. Craig got up this morning and went running since I didn't need to be to the store until 10:00. He ran for about an hour and a half and found his way home with help. He tells me he always sees people that he knows and talks to them and that I know them. I have no idea who he is ever talking about. I brought him home some lunch and he is always happy to see me. He said he was tired from running and he just wanted to rest. I always remember the thought that before you leave this earth you sleep a lot preparing for your final journey. He went over to visit with Suzanne and the children this afternoon and went for a walk around the block with Suzanne and Sigmund (their dog). I got him in the tub tonight and let him soak after his sleeping pills. He all but fell asleep in the tub, then got out and wanted "doast," which I reminded him he had before he got into the tub. Then he inquired about his Tylenol, Vitamin E and garlic pill. He's got a routine of everything he thinks he needs. He has no idea when he takes them or if he takes them. He still tells people that he takes two little white pills every day and I don't even give him aspirin any more. He takes no little white pills.

I put a plastic mattress cover under the sheet and it came loose in the night. He said you know that no matter who I slept with (dreamt about) I was in a tin shed. The plastic sounded like tin to him. He wanted to know if I heard it or if it was rain. It took me until I made the bed to figure out what he was talking about. I put the plastic under the mattress cover so he wouldn't hear or feel the plastic and we'll just have to figure out the mattress pad with the sheets. I finally found one at a medical supply store that is waterproof.

I just wish that life was a lot simpler, but I don't know if I could handle it any better. I've come to the conclusion that by being busy I remain sane and happy. Some days I feel very anxious inside and some days I feel like I can handle anything. I'm more at peace with most every aspect of it all now and hopefully, I am prepared for whatever is next.

March 22, 1998. *"With faith all things are possible and with love it makes it easier"* — Craig talked to Mark and Paul today. He loved both of these guys so it made him very happy to talk to them. He rattles on with them and tells them stories they've each heard a million times. I love them both for being so kind to him. I pray for continued peace. It's been a hard day. I got called to work twice today. I feel like I could just sit by myself and cry tonight. My throat feels sore and I feel sad tonight. I also am mixed up about what is happening about the store. I almost wonder if my sore throat isn't the smoke at the store and we're thinking that is what Stephen may be suffering from (allergies/smoke). Craig talked to the people at church today about "volunteering" at The Alzheimer's Center. I told him Heavenly Father likes it when we volunteer and not take pay. One of the hardest things at night is to sit here and have him talk on and keep repeating the same stories over and over and constantly wanting me to call someone for him. It's great when the pills start to work and he gets heavy eyelids.

March 23, 1998. *"Find an aim in life before you run out of ammunition"* — Craig got up early (6:00) this morning and wanted to run. He ran for two and a half hours, got back—I don't know how. He had a bad accident and was bloody. I still can't figure out the blood. I got him cleaned up and in the shower and literally had to scrub him down today. He was terribly confused today. He went to visit his mother for a few hours. I know that he has asked me the same question at least 15 times now.

March 24, 1998. *"Never doubt yourself"* — I think I have a cold coming on and it doesn't feel very good. Craig went running again today and he's lost his necklace that states he's memory impaired. I found his bracelet and he'll have to wear that until I get him a new necklace. He went and did speed work tonight with Debbie and Karen. They are all so good to him. They made sure he had water and whatever he needs. He can't do many things for himself at all anymore but he still knows us and can converse with people. It's strange. I have no idea how he ever gets home when he can't even figure out how to sit down on the toilet by himself.

March 26, 1998. *"Be a person of value"* — I've had a bad cold and haven't felt well. I took Craig to day care today and went to work for an hour and then came home and slept most of the day. I picked him up at 3:00. He said he didn't like it very much. He played horseshoes with one of the residents and then he said he helped him when he went to the bathroom and can't understand it because he stands to go to the bathroom. He said he liked playing cards with that one lady even though he can't do it very well. I tell him that I "volunteer" there as well. He keeps telling me that I work too hard, that is why I am sick. He tried to tell me he had a sore toe and he had told me 15 times. He had a hole in his sock. I can't figure that one out since all of his socks are pretty new. We threw it away and put on a new one. He also wants me to do away with the doorframes. He said our house is too small and he keeps hurting his knees. Actually it is his elbow that he must have fallen on that the skin is off. He doesn't know when he did it. He doesn't know when he does what any more. He said his dad visited him today while I was at Suzanne's and they have a new drug for Alzheimer's but he didn't know what it was.

Yesterday Craig decided to run. I went to work knowing Suzanne would be right back. She came home and saw him standing in the neighbor's driveway. She asked him what he was doing and he told her that he wanted to tell someone that he was running and I wasn't home and she wasn't home but he didn't think the neighbors were home either so he stood there. Two hours later he came home. Suzanne set his clothes out and turned the water on for him. He got himself dressed. His underclothes were on wrong side out but at least he got them on this time. Last time he didn't remember to put them on. He doesn't know how to sit his cup of hot chocolate down on the coffee table and tries to just hold it. I don't know if it's because he has his sleeping medication starting to work or it just isn't clicking as to what to do.

March 28, 1998. *"Enjoy the day"* — Today was and is a hard day. Craig seems more confused than ever and he seems to know it. This morning he went running and didn't get home before I had to go to work. Suzanne called to say he made it home. She fixed him lunch and helped him dress. I went home at 2:00 and took him something else to eat. He said he didn't like it because it had rocks in it. Anything that is textured or has any substance to it he calls it rocks and spits it out on the table. He had eaten Oreo's and had a big black Oreo smile. It made me smile and I wanted to laugh as he laughed. I think he was just happy that I came home. He had his shirt on with no undershirt underneath and no jeans on. He went over to Suzanne's house and she had a struggle helping him understand to come in and shut the door. He started to cry. I knew something was wrong as soon as I saw him and saw his red eyes. Suzanne took him to the store with her and I took the children. Craig wanted to come home, watch Utah basketball on television and have hot chocolate and doast (toast). I have a plant to the side of the television and he said that has to go because he can't see the television with that there. Nothing makes sense any more and he said he couldn't volunteer so much at the Alzheimer's center because his mother is depressed and needs him to come and help her. We had several people that came into the store today and asked about Craig and said many nice things about how helpful, friendly and willing to help everyone he was. Craig is loved by everyone. I have a hard time keeping it together when people ask about him.

March 29, 1998. *"Good intentions are no substitute for action"* — Today has been a long day but I always feel good when I know that I am at home with Craig for the day. I know that is where I want to be. Craig has consented to go to the Alzheimer's Center again tomorrow. I've decided to leave it day-to-day and let decisions be made accordingly. The same with the store. Craig got lost at church today. He was trying to run after someone and let them know something about a person they both know. He moved so fast he was gone before I could turn around. I yelled at Mike and had him help me find him. I got him into bed early tonight. He literally couldn't do anything today.

April 2, 1998. *"In seeking happiness for others, you find it yourself"* — I can't believe the whole week has gone by and I have not written. Craig is more possessive of what I do when I sit by him at night. He said he hates the noise, but I think he doesn't like it when I'm not contributing to his conversations and questions. He went to daycare twice this week and "volunteered." He really likes a fellow named Curt who is close to his age. Curt said he lives there but doesn't like it and can't believe that Craig would volunteer there when he isn't sick. Craig is confused when he helps out there and he sees Curt urinate standing up and he sits down. I tell him some people sit and some people stand. I just know that we have fewer accidents with Craig sitting than standing. He went running tonight when we got home and had another accident. He said that when he got to the park and those places were locked he just took the feces out with his hands and threw it on the lawn and if they weren't going to unlock those places they deserve to clean it up. Besides what do they do with the dog feces? He was almost proud of himself. It makes me frightened if there were people around, especially little children. His behavior is becoming a lot more unpredictable. He talks about his "tinkle" and he comes up with words that I don't know where they are coming from. You can point to a glass and pills on the cupboard and he won't have a clue until you actually put your finger and hand right on the glass and pills. He talked about seeing things last night and then said everyone does that its called stigmatism. I had to figure out the word, stigmatism. He didn't know he was hallucinating. It is getting harder every day and I don't know what to do any more.

April 6, 1998. *"Each day is pay day in labors of love"* — I haven't written since last week because Craig is more obsessed with whatever I do whether it be reading material or whatever. He is very possessive of my time and he chatters on forever. This weekend we went to dinner with Mike and Linda. Craig had a hard time with his hamburger. He has a hard time eating. I think finger food is better and then I think a spoon is better — in reality it is all getting hard. He slipped in the tub tonight and it scared me to death. He said, "It's a good thing I'm such an athlete." His dad picked him up Friday and took him to lunch. Craig got very anxious. He went to the grocery store with me this weekend and insisted on helping. He does not know how to pick up bags and everything falls out of them. When I tell him to just get in the car and I'll do it he becomes very irritated. I almost wish he wouldn't remember some things as well as he does and it would make some things easier. I sometimes wish I knew or could see down the road — perhaps not. He went to lunch with Jesse today. Actually they went for drinks because Craig said he had already eaten with Suzanne. Suzanne said he didn't eat because he said he was supposed to go eat with Jesse. He did know he didn't have any money. Jesse called on the phone and Craig figured out to answer it and then left the phone and said he had to go get his coat and you could hear him trail off — this was on the answering machine. I've noticed too on the phone that he'll say it was nice to see you. I sometimes wonder if he didn't run if his mind wouldn't go even faster than it seems to be. His stories used to be paragraphs, went to sentences and are now just words where you fill in the blanks more than ever.

April 7, 1998. *"Kindness is a language we all understand"* — 9:30 and Craig is in bed. He said he was anxious after a neighbor visited for a while. He had already had a bath and two sleeping pills. I gave him another anti-depressant. Perhaps I should be giving him anti-anxiety instead of anti-depressant's any more. I will feel my way for a little while then talk with the psychologist, a doctor, or the pharmacist about which would be best. Craig went out running by himself again today. I've decided he lets down all barriers when we are home and works hard to keep it together around others. He will not let me help him with his coat if someone is around and he doesn't like to take any pills when anyone is here. It's like: don't tell anyone anything is wrong, even though he tells people he has Alzheimer's or 'Big Al'. It still amazes me that he can differentiate. He won't know to lick an ice cream cone in his hand and at the same time tell you something factual from his very early years. After five or ten minutes of being around him and his compulsive chatter he wears you out. I'm totally exhausted at night but yet my own mind won't turn off. I think because I see the time is getting near to where Craig isn't with me. I anticipate and fear it both at the same time and feel like I am closing a chapter of my life. My heart feels heavy as I venture into this new phase of feeling alone and being alone. My new assignments at work have given me renewed energy along with faxing daily thoughts to Steve. I feel such joy for Steve and Suzanne and their dear mates who I love like my own. They have been such a source of strength and help to me. I know that with faith all things are possible.

April 8, 1998. *"Do one good deed per day"* — Craig is making less sense today. When I turned the corner of our street he was just standing there. I asked him what he was doing and he said he was waiting for the children. They were going to play soccer. He had been sleeping. I know when Suzanne called me she said that she was taking him with her to watch the children play. He said he needed to go sleep, that he was tired. He doesn't understand times anymore. He continues to tell me constantly that I work too much and that's what everyone thinks. He seems to know all of us but there is so much that he can't do and say. Today he roamed from room to room looking for a certain coat and his grandpa's war "thing" because his mom asks him about it. I know his mother doesn't call and ask him about it; but she must have asked about it enough that it is stuck in his mind that she wants it. He has also remembered that his baseball money disappeared. I don't know where it has all come out of lately. These are memories I thought were buried forever. He also told me he was very upset at me when I got home and he couldn't tell me why — he had to show me. There were two rolls of toilet paper on the bed and the roll was empty in the bathroom along with little "brown" marks on the floor. I don't know what happened. The kitchen cupboard was all wet; all the cupboards were open as well as the drawers. I noticed that he ate four cups of pudding. Oh, I can hardly handle all of the chatter tonight. I guess that is what he feels like when I click away on the computer. It brings me some sanity and I know it is therapeutic because I am talking in my own way.

April 9, 1998. *"Love one another"* — I came home at lunch to check on Craig and he was standing in the driveway. He said he was waiting for Jesse to pick him up. He's like a lost child. I gave him some money to put in his pocket. He rummaged through all of the closets today to find a coat he wanted. He said it wore him out because he worked so hard but that I would be proud of him and happy to see what he did. He emptied our closet out. Oh! Now he is obsessed with finding his Grandpa's World War I uniform. He said his mom wants to know where it is. He picks up little pieces of lint or dirt from the floor and said he likes things clean. Oh, he has no idea. He ate all of his dinner tonight. I made him chicken. He always picks little pieces out and puts them on the table to the side of his dish and says they are rocks. When the sleeping pills start to work he doesn't talk as much. Bill called tonight to talk to him. He gets confused as to how to hold the phone and he will constantly look at me and talk to me instead of into the phone. I end up holding the phone and sometimes telling him what to say.

April 10, 1998. *"Let there be peace on earth and let it begin with me"* — Today was a busy day. I got up early and went in to work before 7:00 to get ready for a meeting and then came home before Craig woke up and got breakfast and myself ready then got him taken care of for the morning. He's looking forward to watching the Master's Golf Tournament on television. It got rained out or rain delayed so he decided to go running. He asked the people up the street to watch for him and he said they must have forgot because they weren't here when he came back home, which was a good thing because he had another accident. But this time he was going to be smarter than Big Al - he smashed it. He couldn't explain to me how he did it so I just told him I understood and laughed with him. He thought he was pretty smart. When I came home today he was standing with only a towel around him. He had tried to wash his shorts out and thought he had lost his ID necklace. He had left it at Suzanne's. He thought he was sick and hadn't eaten for the day. I reminded him that he ate with Suzanne and he didn't think he had or if he did it wasn't enough. I know that he had $1 in his pants pocket and he said Suzanne needed it. He thought she spent all of his money. I need to make sure that he has his own money to use or not use so he feels in control. He said he didn't feel good. I helped him get dressed and then we had bread/butter and soup. He ate it all and then started to cry and say he didn't feel good and something wasn't right. He hoped he would feel better before he went to see the doctor. I held him and he cried and I reassured him that it was all right. I took him by the hand and said let's go get in a hot tub. I thought that would relax him. I gave him his sleeping pill and let him soak for ten minutes that got him out and rubbed him all over with lotion and made him some hot chocolate. There was an advertisement on television about legs and he thought something was wrong with the television or his eyes that he couldn't see their whole body. Then there was a talk show and one fellow kept using his hands when he talked. Craig thought there was something wrong with that and became obsessed when he would see this guy's fingers. He's amazed that we can see things from New York or anywhere in our house. Telephones amaze him as well. Tonight when I put him to bed he called me by name, Judy, which he hasn't done for a long time and told me thank you and that he loved me. It was like the old Craig was in there. I told him he didn't ever need to thank me but he was welcome and if I was the sick one he would be helping me and that I loved him too. It made my heart happy and sad. Oh, he's declining. I've slept on the couch for the past few nights — I don't know why because I actually feel more alone down here than in the bedroom next to him. I've got to go to work at the store tomorrow so I better try to sleep.

April 11-12, 1998. *"You are not responsible for your heritage, but you are responsible for your future"* — It has been a long weekend. I worked at the store all day on Saturday. I went home to get Craig and he had gotten in a shower by himself and was partially dressed. I told him we were going to go to Steve and Wendy's to take the girls an Easter book and present to have on Easter morning. That made him happy. We only stayed a short time and then came home and had hot chocolate and went to bed so we could get up early this morning for Craig to run with his friends. I woke him up at 6:15 and it was still dark. I turned the light on and told him it was time to wake up. He said he had a hole again and it's all wet. I don't know if he is so sleepy from the pills or he just doesn't know to get up because it seems to happen almost every night. I've tried to limit the amount of liquid at night any more. He had an erection when he got up and he got this surprised look on his face and said, "Oh, my gosh look — what's wrong—I've never seen it look like that." I tried to reassure him that it was all right and to just get up so we could hurry to get dressed for running and it would be all right. Pretty soon he felt better and things were normal again. He was pretty animated today. He goes on and on and never quite takes a breath. They laugh a lot so he just keeps going on and on—almost like the Everyready Bunny. I've got to visit a medical supply place tomorrow and get some sheets for the bed and pants for Craig to wear at night.

April 16, 1998. *"God comforts us, not to make us comfortable, but to make us comforters"* — Today was a good day. I had a great day with Steve. He taught me how to play darts and we talked one-on-one for probably two hours. He took me to see his rental house and new garage they are building for his trailers and trucks. I told him that we are indeed blessed to have somebody so wonderful for so long. He asked me about his funeral and if he was going to speak. I told him all three of us were. I told him we haven't lost him yet. We both agreed that in some ways it would be nice to be tomorrow and in other ways you want it never to come. I believe Steve wanted to be able to take his dad hunting and say good-bye and Craig was too anxious and nervous at that time to go away. Steve is going to care for his dad when I go to New York next month. When I got Craig up this morning he had no clothes on. He said look what happened — if you wouldn't give me clothes with holes this wouldn't happen. All of the drawers were open and everything out of them. I've been sleeping on the couch in the family room the past week and I didn't hear him in the night. Bad & good — good in that I sleep better. He went to lunch with Richard and Bob today. When I got home he wanted to go running. He was the most confused about putting the right clothes on. He only wanted shorts because it was warm and then he wondered about putting his gaiter and gloves on. I got him in the tub and let him eat his dinner while I went to pick up the laundry. He ate everything on his plate and was still sitting at the table when I got back and his hands were greasy from picking up the fish and the fries. He said look at me - I made a mess. I just smiled at him and said he wasn't a mess, that's what happens when we eat food we have to pick up with our fingers, gave him a napkin, then had him run his hands under hot water and dried them. He'll run them under the hot water but doesn't know what to do with the towel to dry them off.

April 19, 1998. *"Today I will be the kind of friend that I want others to be to me"* — I'm sitting here alone in the dark tonight with a feeling of aloneness. Craig seems rational at times and I talk to him like a person with no dementia and realize I am trying to rationalize with an irrational person. He became angry today stating that I work too much. I finally got so tired of hearing it that I said that because I wasn't sick I couldn't retire. He became even more upset. I was trying but to no avail. We went for a ride to Su's and visited with her and her mother. She is great to just sit and listen to him. It's becoming more wearing each day: Craig, the store and the day-to-day of preparing for the next day. Work is my only source of relief or refuge. He's slipping away. I'm prepared, but I'm not. I'm prepared for him to die and pass on, but I'm not prepared to put him in a nursing home. He keeps telling me that one lady out there tells him he is handsome. I'll have to figure out which lady it is and tell her I agree. He had a hard time with words today — they just would not come together. I try not to do things for him that I know he can still do. We pulled into the driveway and I waited for him to open the car door and then realized he didn't know how and when I opened it up for him, he said, 'well, you sure are a butt-hole' – I've not heard Craig talk to me like this and I just looked back at him and told him 'that he was a butt-hole too' – When I put him to bed and tucked him in I told him I loved him and he looked up at me and told me he was sorry for saying that and I apologized too. He said Heavenly Father doesn't like me when I talk like that and I assured him he didn't like either of us to talk like that.

April 21, 1998. *"Love through actions"* — Craig "volunteered" today. This morning he was getting out of the shower and had a bowel movement just standing there. He knew it was wrong and apologized, but he just doesn't understand to move to the toilet. He told someone at the Alzheimer's Center today that if his name was there by a bed in the 'motel' part that meant he was staying but he didn't know for how long. He's still got some things figured out. He also knows they have their names on their clothes and glad he only has Nike on his clothes and not his name. He went over to the track tonight and ran with Debbie, Jeanne and Karen. He was very tired, ate and got in the tub. He was so tired and confused that it wasn't too hard to get him to bed tonight. He is so repetitive that it makes it harder at night to sit and watch television with him. We talked to Steve on the way to the center this morning. I told him that Steve volunteers there too. I don't quite know how to handle the prospect of him staying there for a week. But, I also know it is the only way to go and not worry about someone caring for him.

April 23, 1998. *"Always enjoy the beauty of a sunrise and sunset"* — It has been two days of hell for both of us. Craig went running yesterday and came home and I don't know what happened from there. Suzanne called me at work to prepare me for the smell. She opened all the windows and our carpet in the bedroom that is off-white is brown. There were feces everywhere. He tried to clean it up. It was on the bed, on the dirty clothes in the hamper, on the wall, all over the bathroom walls, rugs, shower curtain, toilet and tub. I went for a ride, went to the store, came home and scrubbed for the third time and disinfected everything. Today I came home to almost the same thing. I can't get it out of the bedroom carpet and today I had to throw away the bathroom rugs and shower curtain. It was all over the bathroom walls as well. He had three undershirts on and one shirt on top of those. He felt bad and knew he had done wrong. I try to say everything is okay, but I'm sure he knows better. I got him in a hot tub tonight, scrubbed everything down again, cut his fingernails and shaved him with the electric razor thinking it would relax him. It's the third night with the new sleeping aid. I hope it works tonight and knocks him out until tomorrow morning. I haven't slept well myself for the last two nights but mostly because of my own sore throat. I think I've just let myself get a little stressed wondering what to do anymore day-to-day. I know if I could stay home everyday and protect him, watch over him every-day, he could do a lot better. I don't know if I could handle seven days without being away though. Alex and Emily told me that the reason I'm smarter than grandpa is that I am older than he is and that pretty soon he is going to start wearing diapers like Jamison. Suzanne told me that they all saw the mess on the floor so she tried to explain even more of "grandpa's" illness. I bought a book through the Alzheimer's Association, *Grandpa Doesn't Know Me Anymore*.

April 24, 1998. *"Make the best of what you have because you can't always have the best"* — Craig slept until almost 8:00 today and then wanted to go volunteer (but just for half-day). I really think he feels like he's helping people. He told me today that this one person just got left there and then he said, "You wouldn't do that to me would you?" I don't know how I'm going to handle the week I go away. It's coming soon. He is very upset about the stain still on the bedroom floor so I went and got a throw rug to put over it so he wouldn't see it. The days are definitely getting harder. They are finally starting to rebuild at the store since the fire and it looks like we're closed. So, business is definitely slow. I can't believe how mixed-up Craig is becoming. He came home and wanted to change and go running. He didn't know how to lace and tie one shoe and yet got the other one on okay. He then took the shoes back off and his shorts and said he had gas. He went and used the bathroom and didn't know where his clothes were and they were on the floor right in front of him. This is one strange disease. If we think the body is miraculous — imagine the brain and all the neuro transmitters. I really believe that if I didn't drill it into his head every day that he wasn't getting worse that he might have tried to take his own life. Now I don't think he would know how. He wanted to kneel down and say his prayers and when we knelt down instead of kneeling, he bent over on all fours and that is how we said our prayers. After that I always tried to have him lying down in bed to say prayers.

April 26, 1998. *"Keep a prayer in your heart"* — It's 10:00 and Craig is in bed. He somehow seemed coherent tonight before he went to bed. He bumped his elbow again on the doorframe and it didn't seem to bother him as much as it usually does. He did repeat the phrase that "when is Steve going to come and fix these things?" He also looked at the clock on the nightstand and it said 9:15. He said it isn't 10:00 it's only 9:00. I was dumbfounded that he knew that. I always tell him the news is over and it's after 10:00 and time to go to bed. I know that I'll be so alone when he is no longer here but right now I feel peace when he's in bed. He's more confused but almost seemed like some of him was here off and on today. We went out to visit Steve, Wendy and the girls tonight. Taylor and Madison are so cute. We waited for Wendy and the girls to come home from church and then we went with them to feed some horses up by their church. The children loved it and it was fun to be with them. I miss being able to have the children around more, but Craig does better when there is little or no confusion. He struggles more and more at putting on clothes and taking them off.

April 29, 1998. *"Giving and forgiving are what makes life"* — Craig wanted to go volunteer today. I think it makes him feel good to be around people all day chatting away. He wanted to play golf yesterday and went to Suzanne's to tell her he was going. She called Steve to come pick him up and they went to hit balls. When Steve came to pick him up he had no pants on and two different shoes on the wrong feet. He said he knew something was missing. Yesterday he had on two pairs of Levi's. He told me his dinky felt funny and I assumed he didn't have any underpants on. I was shocked to see he had two pairs of Levi's on. I don't know how he accomplished that one. He has a hard time putting one pair on. He went for another run today when we got home. He was tired when he came home and he had a long bath before eating and then we watched television until bedtime. He wants things to have one hole versus two so it would be easier (his shorts). I told him everyone had two because we have two legs. Tonight he wanted to do that thing that made his mouth feel good — brush his teeth. And asks, "Where did we get that good stuff?" Even at wiping his hands off he is always amazed when I help him with something and it's so easy for "me" and he just can't understand I know how to do those things. He is definitely a sweet and gentle spirit – much like a little child.

May 2, 1998. *"Prayer is an armor — don't go into the day without it"* — We had a yard sale today (mostly Suzanne) but I brought a bunch of things from the store. Business has been incredibly slow since the fire. They have so much construction going on that it looks like we are out of business. We ended up selling close to $700 of store stuff and almost $1,000 for Suzanne. Craig spent most of the day just hanging around and "helping" — it was a great day. I love my family. I got Craig dressed and let him go running. It makes a big difference when I'm around. A woman whose husband has Alzheimer's came to the sale today. She and Craig talked and I told him that she and her husband volunteer there as well and that he stays overnight once in a while. Craig got this look on his face — not me. He wants so much to help and he tried to help pick up afterwards and is not coordinated at all. He doesn't know how to pick up a table to move it and he doesn't understand that he doesn't know what to do. The mind and how it ceases to function amazes me. Some days he can't undress himself and becomes confused. He tries to take his pants off without taking his shoes off first...just little things. Yesterday he put on his undershorts and shirt and then tucked his shirt in his underpants and put on his shoes and socks, knew something was wrong but didn't know what. I told him he didn't have any pants on and he needed to take his shoes off, put his jeans on and then put his shoes back on. He's becoming more confused with his stories he tells as well. I don't know what he will say when I tell him he's going to a Jazz game tomorrow with Steve. Pat called tonight to check on things. They are such good friends. They love Craig.

May 4, 1998. *"When God measures a man — he puts the tape around the heart instead of the head"* — Steve and Wendy took Craig to the Jazz playoff game yesterday. I had been given box seats. They had food, drinks and their own restroom in the box. All three of them had a good time. Craig really liked it. I stayed at home and played with Taylor and Madison. We had fun playing house, games, watching "Annie" and going for hot dogs. We went to feed carrots to the horses and got ice cream with M&M's. All in all it was a great day where we all had a good time. Craig seems more confused today. He doesn't know how to take his own pants off and keeps saying his head hurts so bad that his ears are moving. He's struggling about where to put his legs into his jeans. Steve said it best about his language skills. It's like he's speaking a different language. He goes on and on about something and you have no idea what he is talking about. I feel like I'm the only one that knows what is going on in his mind and only because I've heard the story a dozen times or more. I'm going to try to have him volunteer tomorrow.

May 5, 1998. *"Never borrow from the future"* — Craig volunteered again today at the "Alzheimer's Center" — He slept until almost 9:00 this morning. He seems to be comfortable once we get there. He enjoys listening to the radio in the car. He is still obsessed that the people at the center don't have vitamin E. I told him they take it with their breakfast before he gets there and they just forget. He likes the people there. He talks a lot about a woman that plays cards with him that is in a wheelchair and a gentleman who must have been a potato farmer because he talks about him needing to go home and harvest his potatoes and apples. He said he would bring Craig some if he would help him get home. He ran with Karen tonight. She is great with him. He calls her Carol and neither one of us correct him. Her children are kind to him as well. He had a little accident in his pants again. He smelled and he couldn't figure out what was wrong. He kept saying it was just gas. I just assure him that everything is okay. I talked to Steve and Suzanne today about taking care of him while I go to New York next weekend. I'll be glad to go but probably glad to be back even before I go. It will be so nice to take baths and not worry about hurrying and getting dressed up and going out and being able to relax for a day.

May 6, 1998. *"Smile – God loves you"* — Craig slept late today. I went to work early, came home and he was still in bed. It was a great start to the day. Perhaps because it was raining it appeared darker. I went back to work tonight for a while so he fell asleep earlier because I wasn't here to chat with. He went running tonight when I got home from work. He was very agitated that someone stopped and asked him if I knew where he was. He told them that he didn't have Alzheimer's anymore. He went to a clinic and now he can run every day. I'm appreciative that people watch over him when he's out. He came home again with his pants full. I don't know how he ever comes back home like that. It's got to be miserable. This was the hardest one for me to clean up. He actually forgot he got in the tub after he ate and was tired and asked to get in the tub again. Suzanne took him up to his mother's for lunch today. She stayed with them and then brought him home. Craig said his mother is going to get a new car and he can't believe that because she's too old to drive. He said, "I think she must be 90." Tricia called to check on Craig and see how he was doing. She misses seeing him at the cleaners. He would always go in and make them laugh with his stories. Their whole family are wonderful friends.

May 7, 1998. *"Be humble"* — I left Craig home today. He had lunch with Suzanne but mostly stayed at home. He said he was tired of running for a while. He is so talkative tonight and I think it is because he has been home alone today. He has been talking non-stop. He seems to talk better tonight. He even ate better tonight with less mess. He did have water all over the kitchen counter and floor. He turns the waterspout to run on the counter instead of the sink. I try to leave him a drink container full and a dish of pretzels, crackers and a granola bar when I leave each day. I pray that he could go while he has dignity and his grandchildren know him the way he is instead of in a care facility. He was still upset this morning over someone stopping him yesterday when he was running and asked him if I knew where he was. He said he just went to see the doctor at the clinic and takes two pills and is okay and won't ever get any worse. He said he wanted to tell her that he ran every day and knows every route in Provo. He did better at getting in and out of the tub tonight. It seems to relax him and it is an easier way to get his hair shampooed and his body all scrubbed off.

May 8, 1998. *"Be sincerely interested in others"* — Another hard day. It started off with Craig taking the drawers out trying to find his favorite white running shirt. I had no idea which shirt or where it was and I told him I would help him when I got home after work. He told me tonight that he found it. He watched videos today and Suzanne fixed him lunch. Craig said he got lonely today. It made both Suzanne and I sad. He wanted to go running even though it was raining hard. I think he just wanted to be out. We had soup and a bath and watched television together before falling asleep. He came up and tapped me on the shoulder while I was doing the dishes and said he was sorry for getting mad at me. It breaks your heart. This interim period before graduation is tough. I just want him to be able to have his dignity when he leaves. I want to be able to cuddle up with him at night, snuggle and hold him in my arms forever.

May 10, 1998. *"The greatest gift a father can give to his children is to love their mother"* — Mother's Day and perhaps our last: the last being where Craig knows us. We went to brunch with Steve, Wendy and the girls today. Steve took care of his dad and told me to relax and just take care of me. Craig is always confused by the amount he does for him. Craig thinks he can do all of these things himself. We had a great time and the food was wonderful. They gave me a print that Steve picked out himself. I loved it. Suzanne came over and gave me a beautiful card with a sweet sentiment. She has invited me to a play tomorrow night and arranged for Craig's mother to take him for the evening. My children have been wonderful and very supportive. I talked to each of my sisters over the past two days. It was nice to talk to them. I sent a note to Gladys recognizing the fact that God placed us on this earth as mother and child and thanked her for being my mother and that I prayed that God would bless her. Craig wished me a happy mother's day and said he loved me. He even asked for a kiss. I think this was my last Mother's Day with Craig and my heart aches tonight and my eyes are filled with tears.

May 11, 1998. *"A few simple elements combined in a proper way form a sturdy foundation"* — The day started off with Craig trying to find clubs and he couldn't find his driver. Needless to say I never know where anything is anymore. Bill picked him up and took him to hit balls. He was pretty excited. He spent the evening with his mother. Suzanne took me to a play in Salt Lake for my Mother's Day present. It was fun to spend time with her and just chat. We went to get a quick bite and then to the theatre for the play. We talked about Craig and laughed at some of the funny things he does. Last night when he went to bed he told me he was going to talk and when I asked him who to - he said Heavenly Father and you could hear him just talking away. The last few days he has called Taylor, Tay-Tay, and Madison, Medison. He adores the children. They are definitely the jewels in his crown. Suzanne said when she checked on him today he was washing his golf balls in the toilet. He told her they were dirty. I think he doesn't know how to turn the water on in the sink and so the toilet bowl was filled with water. She said Alex is concerned he's going to get worms because he doesn't wash his hands after he uses the bathroom. Actually, he's pretty good about washing his hands; he just doesn't know how to dry them. I try to have the waterless soap that pumps out. Pat and Tricia both called me tonight to encourage me along and check on Craig.

May 12, 1998. *"Learn and experience the wonders of life"* — Craig volunteered again today. Each time he goes he says it is his last and only for a half. Each morning when I have him sit on the toilet to shave him we talk about volunteering. Some days he wants to go and some days he doesn't. On the days he says it is my turn I will tell him that I volunteered yesterday and today is his turn. He sits there for a minute and asks me if I'm sure and then he says, 'oh, okay but you better be on time.' Today when I picked him up I took him back to the office to meet some new people at work. I think he had a good time. It makes him feel like he's among his old friends. I work with some pretty neat people. Craig got up before 7:00 this morning, which was a little, strange since we didn't get to bed until 12:30 last night and he usually goes around 9 or 10. I told him he had to go back to bed because it was too early to get up and he said he would but he needed my help. He had no bottoms on. I never could find them. The only thing I can figure out is they are flushed down the toilet because I heard the toilet flush 2-3 times. They must have had him stand to urinate today and he had a little accident because they washed and dried his clothes and said they needed to get it done before his wife picked him up. He told me his dinky felt funny and there was something wrong. When we got home and he said "good, now I can use the bathroom the right way." — sitting down to urinate, he had on a pair of jockey shorts underneath his own and then his jeans and socks that had someone's initials on and his shoes had been redone. He also said he didn't like that one guy very well and the food was yucky today. They told him it would be better tomorrow.

May 14, 1998. *"What we become will be what we prepare for now"* — It is the night before I leave to go to New York and I'm excited and nervous. I'll tell Craig tomorrow morning that I am going to Park City for two days. Airplanes frighten him so I won't tell him I'm flying anywhere. He went running again tonight and had another accident. I told Suzanne not to let him run while I am away. She promised to keep him busy. He is still looking for his golf club and I do not know where it is (his driver and Big Bertha). He went to lunch with Richard and Bob today. He told me they went to lunch at the store. It took me a long time to figure out that the store was the golf course. It is becoming more and more like a foreign language. It should be interesting to come home after five days and see how he is after being away.

May 22, 1998. *"Express your gratitude"* — I went to New York for five days. I had a wonderful time. I kept busy going to Bar Mitzvah festivities and work meetings. I found time to go to church on Sunday and there was a parade in downtown celebrating the 50th year of statehood for Israel. I called home on Monday night to tell Craig I would be home the next day. He said he didn't remember me saying good-bye so he thought maybe we were getting divorced. I'm sure it was hard for Steve to tend his dad for four nights. Suzanne helped get him ready for church along with her three children. She amazes me. I have a hard time getting just him dressed. He said I was going to be upset because Steve had made a mess after I just cleaned so good. There was some popcorn on the floor by the garbage can. Anything on the floor is upsetting to him lately. He told me he had fun playing darts with Steve and Carl. I wondered why the picture that was hanging above the mantle was sitting on the floor. He volunteered today and said this one lady scares him because she said he is handsome. I let him run tonight and he came home with no accidents in his pants. After I got him in the tub and we had dinner we watched television. I put my feet up on the couch and he asked me what those were. I told him my feet and he said they were the ugliest things he had ever seen and I should get me some new ones. Did everyone have them? He wanted to know if my relatives had them that ugly. He also asked if he had feet too and if he did, were they as ugly as mine. It was all I could do to not laugh. I've noticed that he calls Suzanne Judy a lot. I don't know if it is the week I was away or it is just part of the disease. My nephew committed suicide while I was away. I need to deal with that now and see what I can do to help with the healing process. I don't tell Craig anything that goes on around us. We just deal with his world everyday.

May 23, 1998. *"It is better to appreciate the things you don't own than to own things you don't appreciate"* — Craig slept until 8:00, got up, ate breakfast and went running. I'm forever amazed when he walks through the door. A neighbor, 15, took him to hit balls and they played the executive course at East Bay. Both of them loved it. I watched him hit the ball and he had a hard time making contact. Craig used to be a two handicapper. He would forget to pick up his golf bag and sometimes pick it up and all the clubs would fall out. It took them over two hours to play the executive course. We all went for a late lunch of hamburgers, fries and sodas. It was nice to spend some time away because I was really struggling today. I don't know if it was being able to be away from it or because he seems to be declining and much more repetitive. We went for a walk with Jamison and stopped by to visit some neighbors. It was nice to be with others to listen to him and fill in the blanks. He almost got upset when I got Jamison in the tub before him. We got all settled and then remembered that I hadn't fed Craig any dinner since we ate a late lunch. He seems to take a long time to eat. I got him to go to bed early because I think he was tired and he's going to get up early to run with Bob and Richard early tomorrow.

May 26, 1998. *"Have an attitude of gratitude"* — Craig volunteered today. I picked him up early so he could go run with Karen and Debbie at the track. He fell down and scraped his knees, elbow and hands. He did a pretty good number on himself. Yesterday he went and came home twice with little accidents in his pants. He can't understand what he does wrong he says when he does everything perfect. He said, "I may as well kill myself if I can't run because what else is there." I don't think he could do anything to himself because I don't think he would know how to carry anything out. He seems to get more upset with me when I try to help him out and yet expects me to help him. He is the same when I try to help him get in the car and assist with his seat belt. He can't do it by himself yet thinks he can and seems to get upset when it isn't done. His Big Bertha club is lost or missing and he wouldn't let up on it so I bought a used one and Steve had it reshafted for him. It has a totally different head but he doesn't know. He just thinks it is refinished—I guess. Now, we have to come up with a white shirt that he thinks is missing for running.

May 27, 1998. *"Be a faithful servant"* — I worked at the store tonight and Craig had dinner with Suzanne. I called before I came home to see if anything was needed and he said he wanted those things that make you sleep. After a little questioning we figured he wanted onion rings. He ate the whole order by himself. Suzanne said they had waffles and he wanted an onion with it. She said that one night for dinner while I was away they made hamburgers and she sliced an onion and he ate every slice, but not on his hamburger. He would probably eat it like an apple if I had them around. He's got it in his head that they are good for you and they make you sleep well. He used to hate onions. This morning before I left I sat out some pudding for him. He relates pudding to "Coon" — a friend who he saw eating some one day. He calls it tubbins or something. He can't get the top off by himself and I wanted to help him. He wouldn't let me. Tonight he told me that he loved me and that he knew that with his disease he needed help from people. He said he sat on the floor and cried this morning and asked Heavenly Father for help and pretty soon he was able to open the pudding. When I put him to bed he told me he loved me again. He has such a good heart. He talked to Steve tonight about going golfing together. Craig said that would be such fun to be together. This is September at the time of the St. George Marathon. He seems to be more confused each day.

May 28, 1999. *"Contentment comes not from getting what you want but from enjoying what you have"* — He 'volunteered' today and Susie picked him up for lunch. She took him for burritos and to Squaw Peak for a ride. He told me later they had great pizza and went to see the eagles. She had taken him earlier to Squaw Peak and he wouldn't get out of the car, thinking he would fall off the cliff. This time he got out and they talked about the birds and the eagles. She told him they couldn't get close to the edge because they couldn't fly like the eagles and he agreed. I called a neighbor one morning this past spring that Craig likes and asked him if he could pick Craig up and take him for a ride. They went to see eagles up Springville Canyon. I'm sure that came back to him when he and Suzie went to Squaw Peak and saw birds.

May 30, 1998. *"Do not follow where the path may lead, go instead where there is no path and leave a trail"* — Today is a day of confusion. I've not felt good for the past week and the last two days I've had no energy. I can't afford to be sick and take care of Craig. He keeps calling Suzanne me and me Suzanne. He went running today and someone told him to be careful because he could die and it upset him and told whoever it was that everybody is going to die. He's appreciative of the things you do for him. He's struggled with his food and pills. He has a harder time putting it all together and how to do it.

May 31, 1998. *"The greatest work you do is within the four walls of your home"* — I stayed home today and had Mike take Craig to church. He went running with Bob, Richard and Ed early this morning. Richard brought him home and told me his mother died this past week of Alzheimer's. Her bowels ruptured. Suzanne said last week when he was looking at a book he saw a woman with a necklace and thought she had Alzheimer's because it looked liked his necklace. His Lost Program ID. He even thought she was cute. Susie took him for a ride this afternoon to visit the gravesites and pick up the flowers from Memorial Day. Craig enjoys spending time with her. He's concerned with me not feeling good and so wants to help. When he takes his ID necklace off he calls it his glasses — "here, take my glasses." Suzanne stopped by to see if we wanted to walk around the block and he had to get dressed because he had just gotten out of the tub. I tried to talk him out of it and he got upset and I had to talk him out of being mad and just getting dressed. It's worse than a child is because there is no reasoning. It is definitely a challenging disease. I thought I would have problems getting him to go to bed now that it is light so late, but once he starts falling asleep and is tired he'll usually go to bed thinking that I am going to bed too.

June 2, 1998. *"Tell your loved ones that you love them – life is short – don't let these moments escape you"* — Craig volunteered today. He gave me a kiss as we walked out the door and said he deserved two kisses. I told him he could have as many kisses as he wanted. Sometimes his comments take me so off guard. I try to stay on my toes to always be positive with him and I try never to let down and cry in front of him as though anything were wrong. These past days he seems more confused. Suzanne asked if I would pick Emily up from pre-school today. I picked her up first and she went in with me when I picked Craig up. He was excited to see her, but I think she was a little nervous with all of the elderly people there. Craig seemed to enjoy it more today and said he even liked the food. He had to go to the bathroom and could hardly wait for us to get home. He was either very anxious or more confused but he did not know how to get out of the car and he bumped his head, took his shoes off and as I tried to help him he just said I made him mad. I went in the house ahead of him to turn the bathroom light on for him and make sure he was okay then I took Emily home. It's pretty good when I have to take care of Craig's needs ahead of a little child's. That says a lot. He went running at the track tonight and they said he kept veering to the left as he ran. I think it's that he doesn't know how to navigate the turns very well and he overcompensates as he rounds the bends of the track. It took probably 30 minutes to eat his sandwich. It is taking him longer to eat and do most things. He got in the tub and he keeps saying there are rocks. Every little rough spot he thinks is a rock and he constantly picks things up from the rugs and says it is a rock even if it is a piece of lint or something. It's hard when the children four and five appear to know more than he does. We went to dinner with the children last night and they correct him. It breaks my heart to see the decline. I wish he could sometimes go quickly while he is still "Craig" — the person he was and would like to still be. Except this Craig has taught a lot of people a lot of things about life and living and the importance of each day. Craig made a funny statement on our way to volunteer today. He said we should move to a new place instead of living where everything is old and war stuff. Craig has never wanted to leave this house. I don't think I could move right now while he has familiar things around him especially the neighborhood where people know him and he can go running around the area and he'll get back home. Our friend, Su, that talks to him a lot at night said she enjoys listening to him. She took a class once on listening and it is good practice because in order to fill in the blanks you have to really listen to him. That's exactly right...you can't tune him out or you won't know how to answer him or even join in the conversation with him. My heart aches for him and I'm starting to feel lost and alone again and that I'm in life alone. There are people around me and I'm still feeling alone. I don't feel comfortable anywhere I sleep anymore and I can hardly wait for morning to come. I love Craig and I so want him to be able to join those loved ones on the other side and yet I still gain so much just having him here with me at night. It is a comfort.

June 3, 1998. *"Reach out to others"* — Today is Susie and Sally's birthday. I never did find either one home this morning. I worked today. Craig stayed home with Suzanne and Jesse took him to lunch. I didn't get to ask much about lunch or where they went. I came home and got him some dinner and talked to Suzanne about giving him his pills and keeping an eye on him. I went to see the Jazz play the Chicago Bulls in the first game of the play-offs. It was fun to spend some one-on- one time with Steve and the game was a good one and the Jazz pulled it off in overtime. A friend of mine gave us box seats. It was a great night out. Craig was in bed when I came home.

June 6, 1998. *"The joy of service is first taught and experienced in the home"* — Craig has had a lot of blood the last few days and says his butt is sore. He didn't want to run today and slept until after 9:30. We went to watch Alex play t-ball and came home and had lunch. I ran a few errands and when I came home he had his jeans on with no underpants and had a little bit of an accident in his jeans. I just can't figure out what happens so many times and in such a short period of time. He was adamant about not wanting to go to his family reunion at Big Rock Candy Mountain. I brought him home some new racing flats and he was so appreciative and loved them — even the flashy color. He said colors don't bother him anymore. I'm anxious to see how he does in his race next Saturday. Crowds make him so anxious and he seems to veer to the left as he runs. He started to talk to Suzanne about sex again today. She told him she didn't want to talk about it anymore with him. They are doing a news short on Normandy and Craig is talking about one of the guys at the Alzheimer's

Center being the one that pees a lot and was in that war. The cars seem to confuse him more than ever at getting in and out and which side to get in and he will talk about not bumping his head. Suzanne and I have got so we just chuckle at listening and watching. It makes him very upset when the children appear to be smarter or they say something that he thinks is teasing.

June 8, 1998. *"Service enriches your life"* — It's late and I'm sitting here with so many feelings inside tonight. Steve called to say they had a great time at the family reunion at Big Rock Candy Mountain and that Grandpa was the oldest brother and he felt bad that none of his children came except his grandson. I'm not surprised but I think the drive was too long for such a short period of time and yet even the time was too long when he would have to stay two nights away in a different place. He's more confused and is so pre-occupied with his butt again. He keeps pulling down his pants to see if everything is okay and he won't have any underwear on or else he examines it to see if it is stained. He's gone through at least three pair today. He seemed to enjoy going to church to celebrate Kelly's missionary homecoming. He ran into an old running friend and enjoyed that. He appears to remember some things so well. I've decided that I want to be able to help others and even though you write something doesn't mean people are going to read it except perhaps the caregiver. No one really understands until they spend extended periods of time with the person including the nights. Bill called tonight to let Craig talk and he would just chatter along. We should have a movie camera rolling as he talks on the phone. No one would or could believe the animation.

June 10, 1998. *"Don't let life crash in on you"* — Oh, the nights are getting longer and tougher. Craig went running tonight for over two hours and went back and forth up the street two or three times. Some friends stopped by and we went out for hamburgers. It was fun and Craig is always a lot of laughs around people anymore because it is like playing charades and he has no inhibitions. He went with his sister today and he said she was nice and had a good time. She wanted him to go to his mother's tomorrow and he said he didn't know if he would or not. He definitely has a mind of his own any more and I have a feeling it will get worse. He had no underclothes on again tonight when I got home. I have no idea what he does with them. He now wants me to arrange for golf lessons again. He never lets things go. It will be interesting after he runs a 10K this weekend because right now he says he has to practice every day for the race. He doesn't understand about getting in and out of the car and doing up his seatbelt. It's getting harder for me to handle the nights as he rambles on and on and keeps asking the same questions over and over. Now he is talking about switching shoes and not running with the Asics. It surprises me how much he does remember. I keep wishing I could have a night of quiet and then I get thinking that I should treasure these days and I'll have a lot of quiet nights and days. Craig has oily skin and I bought an astringent for him and rubbed it on his head tonight. He said it felt good and that a friend told him he was handsome. He said, "That's great do you want a date?" His friend told him "no".

Monday when he went to spend half-day with his mother they got in a wreck. He thinks his mother is 90 and too old to drive. Somebody rear-ended them and totaled her car. Craig yelled, "What the hell are you doing?" It scared her and him. She told him that they don't talk like that. No one is used to Craig swearing. She told him to stay in the car and he said he would do what he wanted and he got out and told the people she was 90 and couldn't drive. They had to wait forever for a policeman to write up a report. He didn't want to go home with her and she dropped him off at our house and the doors were locked. He needed to use the bathroom and was walking up and down the street when one of the neighbors's saw him and took him in and called me. I left work and came home to let him in.

June 12, 1998. *"Don't be afraid to be different"* — Craig keeps complaining that his head hurts and that something happened when his mom was in the accident. He's probably got whiplash but there is no use in taking him to the doctor because he's too confused by questions that people ask him. I don't know how bad his head really hurts or even how well he really sees anymore. He went to lunch with Jesse today. They were going to go for a walk and he said they didn't even though he was telling me about the water and he was frightened when he saw it. He wanted a massage and I couldn't even imagine taking him anywhere — he can't undress and dress by himself and there is no way he would understand about lying on his stomach. I remembered a neighbor and, bless her heart, she is here at our home and giving him a massage. I'm hoping that it will relax him and make him feel better. I'm trying everything I should do to make his life full, but it's hard. Today is a hard day and I've been close to tears. I can't imagine him living for a long time like this and yet he seems so healthy that I can't imagine him going home and graduating. He is so appreciative when you bring him something and do some little thing for him. I think he's anxious and nervous about running in a race tomorrow. He thinks I'm going to sleep in and I keep assuring him that I won't. One Sunday I slept in when he was supposed to run early with his friends and as odd as it is he still remembers. I don't know why I am crying and as strange as it sounds I feel incredibly blessed with so much love and peace in my heart. I feel like Craig is so close to his Heavenly Father that you can feel it most of the time. He tells me that he talks to Heavenly Father a lot and that he mostly asks him to bless others. Perhaps I'm anxious and nervous for him to run tomorrow. I feel like he's this little child that I am to protect and watch over and I'm frightened for him when I am not there to guide and direct him. I hope someday that someone can find out about this insidious disease so that we will know what to do and be able to educate others to help. No one has any idea what goes on because the person looks so normal and Craig has such an athletic physique and is young. When he used to be at the store people asked him if he had a brother, Steve, — our son.

June 13, 1998. *"Life is a gift and what we do with that gift is our gift to God"* — Craig ran his race, Stouffer's, in Springville today. Terry said he did better than he had anticipated but at the end when they were going down a hill instead of kicking it in he let up like he was afraid he was going to fall—probably sensing himself off-balance going down a hill—who will ever know? He had a great time and he gets up early in the morning to run with the Sunday crew. He should be exhausted tomorrow night. We're going to pick the children up at the airport and he'll be excited to do that. Steve called him to tell him he loved him and check on the race before he left to go hunting tonight. Susie came over today and spent the last two hours at the store with me and we had a pizza together. It was fun to visit and relax with each other. We had a few customers to contend with at the last hour but it was nice to spend time together because she loves Craig and appreciates what our life is like. She came home with me and brought him a piece of pizza and I went and got a video for the three of us to watch. It was fun to chat with someone and be entertained with something besides the news. I even had enough together after that to balance my checkbook and get my bills paid. I'm trying to decide if I want to start with the contents of my desk to tackle or wait until tomorrow night. It looks pretty overwhelming — tomorrow night. Craig spilled his hot chocolate down him again tonight and felt bad that he ruined his new shirt he got today. I'm soaking it for the night and hope that it comes clean. I got him in bed and then he decided that he needed to say his prayers on his knees. He got down at the bottom of the bed and kneeled down on all fours and asked Heavenly Father to bless each of the children by name and their parents and for Susie and how kind she is to him. Craig's heart is so good. He is so thoughtful. I love him so very much. I am sad tonight.

June 14, 1998. *"We may not always realize everything we do affects not only our life but touches others too"* — The end of a weekend. We got up early and Craig went running with his friends and out for juice, we went to church, over to Susie's for lunch and then to the airport to pick Suzanne, Alex, Emily and Jamison up from their trip to California and the beach. It is nice to have them home. Stephen stayed in California to help coach at a clinic for the week. I've got a lot of work to do after I get Craig to bed tonight. I try not to do much work while he is up. He doesn't understand and thus doesn't like it when I do work at home. He thinks when I'm typing on the computer that I am working for Novations. He thinks now that he has done his race that he shouldn't run for a while and now he should play golf. This is not going to be an easy summer. Craig likes Sunday because he sees Mike. I'm so very appreciative of the people that are willing to spend time with him. It's like tending a grown up little child that doesn't understand and talks and talks and talks and asks a million questions. I sliced some banana nut bread tonight w/butter and hot chocolate. He remembers that we use to have banana nut bread quite a bit. He keeps talking about his massage and how nice it was. If I could afford I would give him a sleeping pill and have a massage for him every night after I got him to bed. He's also obsessed with having everything "square" — he talks about that when he is running and he is upset about the water knobs in the tub. He must have bumped himself on one of the knobs when he was in the shower or tub or it's that he doesn't know how to turn them off when he showers. He's so pleased when he is able to go to the bathroom by himself. Today at the airport he was very uneasy with all the people. He held on to my arm like a blind person until I asked if he wanted me to hold hands. I went to the bathroom and had him sit on a bench and not move. He said, "wow, there is no way I could go to the bathroom here". I didn't dare get a drink until we got almost home. We went on the moving sidewalk at the airport. It's so unnerving for him to try to get off anything moving. You think he's going to fall and the elevators are just as bad. When we get off you have to tell him this is where we get off and he tells the other people "go ahead" and they are not even getting off. I'm sure people wonder what's wrong.

June 15, 1998. *"Concern yourself with others instead of yourself"* — Craig stayed at home today with Suzanne checking on him. He watched two videos and went to lunch with her and the children. I told her he could volunteer tomorrow. He said he would probably help Suzanne instead. I told him we could decide tomorrow when we wake up and not be so tired. He wants to go watch the other television if it's the same thing because he doesn't like to listen to me on the computer. I had a hard time with him this morning when we got dressed. His underwear had a little hole in the seam and he would not wear it and I had to throw them away and put new ones on him. He went running again and then came home and I had him eat before I got him in the tub. I fixed him a Chimi and it must have been too spicy for him. When I got him out of the tub he said we had to talk and that wasn't his thing to eat and he should have eaten fish. I told him next time I would ask him and we would "communicate" and he said "ya that's the word." So, next time I will make sure I get the standard things to eat. Another person up the street that has Alzheimer's, who is much older than Craig, takes the mail out of their box and throws it away or puts it somewhere and his family can't find it. I told them Craig doesn't even know we get mail and if we did he wouldn't know to go get it out of the mailbox. We went across the street to visit the children for a few minutes and I had him walk with his slippers on. He said he thought we would drive over and when we walked across the street he would stop and pick up sticks or little rocks and throw them, saying they shouldn't be there. He didn't like holding my hand because he felt like I was dragging him along and said just go ahead of me and I will go by myself. That is the reason that I don't take him on too many errands with me and I leave him at home watching television and run quick errands one at a time.

June 16, 1998. *"Giving is the treasure that contentment is made of"* — Craig slept until 8:00 again this morning. I fed him a different kind of cereal this morning and when he got out of the shower he said, "I thought we were going to talk" — I knew he meant communicate and that he wanted his standard cereal — Rice Krispie Treats cereal with a sliced banana. Then I cut his nose a little bit when I was shaving him this morning. I didn't tell him and I just tried to stop the bleeding. He stayed home today and ran errands with Suzanne and the children. He thinks the children don't like him anymore and it makes him sad. I think the children understand more and sometimes ignore him when he talks to them. He's more on their level of understanding or probably less understanding. Anyway it's hard and sometimes it breaks my heart to listen to him. We had dinner with Suzanne and the children and then I went to the store. I was gone longer than I thought and couldn't get Suzanne so I called a neighbor and had him go down and change the channel for Craig until I got home. He thought he wanted money and went and told Suzanne. He was crying when I got home and was sad that he told her to go pay them money because he said she probably didn't have any and he thought we owed them money because they do our yard. He had a real hard time getting out of the tub tonight. He was very confused and it took quite a while to get him out and then he started to cry. It broke my heart. He said he was so upset that he hurt his shoulder. I got him out and gave him a foot, hand and head massage and rubbed his shoulder a little bit. He likes astringents rubbed on his head at night to take away the oily feeling. I held him like a baby tonight while he cried. I wish he could go home. We knelt down to say prayers together tonight and he didn't know how to kneel and we finally just stood by the bed and I put my arm around him and gave him a hug and he said, "I love you Judy." He wants to go volunteer tomorrow. Maybe it makes him feel good to be needed. I've cried myself tonight a lot and my eyes are tired. I'm debating on whether to get up early tomorrow and go into the office before I get Craig up and going.

June 18, 1998. *"Let us all watch over each other"* — Craig volunteered yesterday and had a little accident at the end of the day before I was to pick him up. He said he had to pee so bad that he couldn't wait. He said, "I don't think its pee—it's just wet." I told him that he probably just sat in some water. We went with wet pants to Camille's so he could get his once a month hair cut. It always makes him feel good and she is so kind with him. Steve just got home from bear hunting. Craig is excited to see it. Today Craig went to the golf course for lunch with Richard and Bob. I've cried a lot the last two days because Craig is so sad. It would be so interesting to know what is really going on in his mind. He said the children are smarter than he is. The children know he has Alzheimer's, but they are so young they don't understand everything, especially that we keep everything from him. He seems more scattered than ever. Suzie came over and ate with us tonight. Craig at the end didn't want his cornbread. He remembered that he liked it and wanted it later so he said that he would just take it home with him. I still don't think he caught on that this was his house. He enjoys the foot and hand massages at night and the baby lotion always smells good. He remembers that I put an astringent on his head and because I had just gotten him out of the tub and washed his hair, I didn't put it on. He constantly picks little crumbs or anything on the floor. He still tells me that he loves me when I put him to bed at night.

June 19, 1998. *"Be determined to make a difference"* — Tonight for the first time I feel like Craig is really slipping away. Suzanne told me tonight that they are going to start doing Judy checks instead of Craig checks. He even talked about wearing pads (diapers) tonight. He looked in closets trying to show them to me and tell me he used to wear them. He came home from running with another accident and had had one today as well. He also didn't have an undershirt on when I came home. I don't know what he does because he has such a hard time when I get him dressed each morning. He said, "It's not the disease, Alzheimer's, that makes me do these things, it is just my brain. I need to concentrate more." Oh, if that were only the case. I went to get him a father's day present knowing this may be our last one together. It makes my heart heavy with a knot in the pit of my stomach. Oh, how I wish he could go to sleep and not wake up.

June 20, 1998. *"Be a doer – not a procrastinator – life is short"* — Saturday and it's been a pretty good day. Craig didn't wake up until 9:00 and then he ate and I got him shaved, showered and dressed and he started to cry saying he was dumb and the children didn't like him. He just stood and cried so hard his nose was even running. I just hold him and try to console him. I called Susie and she came over. We stopped by the cleaners and let Craig say hi to Trisha and Kent. He misses his friendship with people that he doesn't see very often any more. We had a fun visit and we got out in the car and Craig spilled a coke all down him so we had to go home and change clothes before we could go to Salt Lake and visit with Bonnie. Joan had company so we just stopped at the mall, had a drink and came home. I went to work at the store for the last three hours of the day. It's always nice to visit with Steve and Terry and catch up on all the running stories. It's my only tie to the store and the race team. I think for the first time today that Bonnie realized how hard it is to be around Craig for any length of time because of his continued repetitiveness. Bill called tonight and is so good to let him rattle on forever. He's actually going to take him to play a few holes of golf this week. That should be interesting. Well tomorrow is Father's Day and I think this will probably be our last one with Craig knowing us. I couldn't bring myself to buy a card because I would be the one to read it to him and I don't think I could without crying. I didn't buy cards for anyone, only for our two Steve's: Steve and Stephen. They are both wonderful dads to our dear grandchildren. We're blessed.

June 21, 1998. *"Parable for Fathers: The young father set his foot on the path of life. 'Is the way long?' he asked. And his guide said, 'yes, and the way is hard. And you will be old before you reach the end of it. But the end will be better than the beginning.' But the young father was happy and would not believe that anything could be better than these years. So he played with his children and grandchildren and the sun shone on them and life was good and the father cried, 'nothing will ever be lovelier than this.' Then came night, and storm, and that path was dark, and the children shook with fear and cold, and the father drew them close and covered them, and the children said, 'oh, dad, we are not afraid for you are near and no harm can come.' And the father said, 'this is better than the brightest day for I have taught my children courage. Today, I have given them strength.' And the next day came strange clouds which darkened the earth – clouds of war and hate and evil and the children groped and* *stumbled and the father said, 'look up, lift your eyes to the light.' And the children looked and saw above the clouds an Everlasting Glory, and it guided them and brought them beyond the darkness. And that night, the father said, 'this is the best day of all, for I have shown my children God.' And the days went on, and the weeks and the months and the years, and the father grew frail, and he was a little bent. But his children were tall and strong and walked with courage. And when the way was hard, they helped their father, and when the way was rough they lifted him, for he was as light as a feather, and at last they came to a hill, and beyond this hill they could see a shining road and golden gates flung wide. And the father said, 'I have reached the end of my journey. And now I know that the end is better than the beginning, for my children can walk alone, and their children after them – my grandchildren.' And the children said, 'you will always walk with us, dad, even when you have gone through the gates.' And they stood and watched him as he went on alone, and the gates closed after him. And they said, 'we cannot see him, but he is with us still. A dad like ours is more than a memory. He is a living presence'. " – Author Unknown* — Father's Day...Craig realized that it was his special day but he said he didn't deserve anything and I told him he did too and gave him a kiss and a hug. I gave him some T-shirts and shorts, Suzanne gave him a shirt and Steve gave him some shorts. I think we all had the same thing in mind. Craig has never worn shorts before he got Alzheimer's even though he has great legs and T-shirts are just easier than shirts with buttons. We all went to eat after church at the Outback Steakhouse. We had a good time together. I'm having a tougher time keeping it together, as he is declining. We went over to Susie's and she rode with us over to put some flowers on our dad's grave. He didn't know where we were and asked about how our dad died and where are we? Cemeteries are almost peaceful to me with the quiet. I know that one day I'll probably dread the silence that I now cherish. These last three days Craig has been totally lost and makes no sense most of the time. Su called tonight. She said her mother is getting closer to death and it scares her a little. She's going to go to the mortuary tomorrow and pick up the papers and I'm going to try to get the Social Security people on the phone. We'll report back tomorrow night about our accomplishments or lack there of. I've already got the packet from the mortuary even though I know I don't need them for a while. I wanted everything done while my head is clear and Craig is still here. I believe Craig senses my shortness and I tell him I'm just tired after he's asked me the same thing ten times in five minutes. He told me just to go to bed and then he asks me to help him go to the bathroom and where he goes and what he should do. Oh!

June 22, 1998. *"Go out of your way to be friendly"* — The beginning of our downhill slide. Craig is starting to hallucinate. Suzanne said she came over today and Craig had had an accident and he was managing the store. I asked if Stephen took him to the store and she said "no" he was managing from home talking and telling imaginary people what he was and wasn't doing. I actually got a diaper on him tonight after he got out of the tub. He thinks they are jockey shorts that he used to wear when he ran with his tights. He said I think they are the things I used to wear. He had no idea. I talked to one of Craig's friends and store patron, a medical doctor, about Craig's medication to sleep. He told me to give him 75-100 mg of Nortriptolene because 300 mg a day is safe. He also gave me the release to get a handicap sticker for the car. I had to get Craig to stand in the shower and squirt him off tonight after he went running. He didn't understand what had happened. He thought it was something that I did. He's also talking about something red and said don't tell Suzanne because she already knows. I have no idea what he is talking about. We had spaghetti tonight for dinner and he wasn't happy about that either. He used to like spaghetti but he said we're supposed to talk before I fix him anything to eat. He wanted a coke and I went to a drive-in and got one for him. I was doing some work tonight while I watched television and he didn't like that and wanted to go to another room to watch television.

June 24, 1998. *Lose yourself in looking out for others and you will find the abundant and gratifying life for yourself"* — Craig volunteered today and it was his choice to go but as always "just for half" — I agreed and off we went. He was crying again this morning and having a hard time. He woke up around 7:30 on his own. He slept pretty well for not having had a sleeping pill. There were a little feces in the bed and his pants that I don't know how it got there on the sheets. He went running again tonight and lasted possibly ten minutes before he came home and had another accident. He kept apologizing and I kept telling him not to worry about it just let's get your clothes off and get in a nice hot tub. I went to the store tonight and bought some new undershorts to try. I also got a 1-800 number tonight that you can special order disposable briefs that would work so much better than the diapers I tried last night. I can't believe that there isn't Depends for grown-ups that are like pull-ups for children. I'm anxious to see and know the price of these briefs tomorrow when I call. I gave Craig two 25 mg Nortriptolynes at dinner and two more at 7:30. Usually when I work on the computer he says he can't stand the noise and goes into the other room. Tonight he said he doesn't care what I do. He reminds me of a sick little child.

June 25, 1998. *"Love wasn't put in your heart to stay – love isn't love 'til you give it away"* — Craig had a hard morning. He first woke up at 6:15 and he never wakes up that early. He said his clothes were all wet. I changed his clothes and had him lay down in a clean bed and he slept until 8:30. He was sad this morning and had muscle reflex twitches really bad. He spilled his juice, his water, lost his pills and didn't know how to get them into his mouth and then drink the water. His cereal he spilled all over and it was a mess this morning. I talked him into going to "volunteer" and thought it would make him feel good to be around others and let him think he was helping someone. He liked the new boxer shorts he wore this morning. And he liked his shorts and T-shirt. He likes to wear one of his oldest pair of shoes that he has and why I don't know. I visited Social Security today and something is wrong with our system. He gets no money for the eight years he spent in the Utah National Guard with six months of it being active duty and Medicare does not cover "custodial" care which is what Craig needs...someone to help him bathe/shower, dress, use the bathroom and eat. My insurance, IHC, covers nothing either. I feel like I have worked my whole life to have it all taken away as I bury the person I love one day at a time as they decline. I think I'll call the doctor tomorrow, make an appointment and have him explain what options I have for Craig as we move forward. I had to go to Salt Lake today so I had Suzanne and the children ride up with me and it was a nice change of pace. I got back to work just long enough to work half day. Visiting Social Security this morning was a half-day of vacation which says a little about how exciting my life is. When I picked Craig up today they were having music therapy and Craig was dancing with one of the aides. He was having fun and said he's just an athlete and should be able to do that because it's like golfing and playing baseball — it's just doing the square. I took his hand and we were walking out when he had the muscle twitches again and he fell to the floor. He jerked my arm, but I didn't say anything I was trying hard to protect his fall. I'm wondering if his equilibrium is off balance since the car accident when his head got jerked. I guess that is why I should go talk to a doctor about this too.

June 28, 1998. *"Spiritual recharging is free"* — It has been a very long day today. We got up early for Craig to run with his friends and he was very confused when I got him up and he was a little angry. After he left I slept until he returned. I haven't felt good the past few days and it feels good to sleep. When he got home he apologized for being mean to me. I let him get in the tub and set there for a while before getting dressed. We didn't go to church this morning and went to breakfast at HobbleCreek with Bill and Doris. We sat and visited for a long time until Sonny came to say "hi." Being around Craig makes a lot of people uncomfortable because they don't know how to treat him. We went for a ride to Payson and Spring Lake and pretty much made a day of it. When we got home we went down to Su's and I let her tell Craig that her mother passed away last night. He just said, "How nice." Oh, if he only knew how nice — or, perhaps he does. One thing for sure is that day by day this is getting harder. I just wish I could get him to go to bed and I could play catch up with my work and then just sit here where it's quiet. I think I feel a loss, too, because I know that Su will move back home to Nevada, which she should. She has been such a support system to me because we understand each other as caretakers. Suzanne is my next and I can't pour my heart out to her because she takes her dad every day and has her own worries as a young mother and wife.

June 29, 1998. *"But they that wait upon the Lord shall renew their strength; they shall mount up with wings as eagles; they shall run, and not be weary, and they shall walk, and not faint." (Isaiah 40:31)* — I have to keep reminding myself that even though Craig is my husband he has become as a child that is sick that I am caring for. And, that I need to find joy in this service. It's hard as he vacillates back and forth. He will tell me thank you for making him hot chocolate and then not know where the bathroom is or how to sit down to use the toilet. I've got to talk to the doctor and get his thoughts and impressions of what I should do next. Also, I need to get a chest x-ray. I want to treat Su to a new outfit for her mother's funeral as my gift to her in lieu of flowers. She has been such a support system and I am truly going to miss her. She wants to come and hang out around Craig as a caretaker for a little bit before she returns home to Nevada and her old stomping grounds. Craig volunteered today and seems to be getting better at it.

July 4, 1998. *"Well done, thou good and faithful servant; thou has been faithful over a few things, I will make thee ruler over many things." (Matthew 25:21)* — I can't believe it's been a week since I've written. It's been a busy and hectic week at work and just plain exhausting. There have been a lot of meetings and Craig seems to be more in left field. He's had a lot of little diarrhea accidents and Thursday morning was pretty bad and as I was cleaning up the kitchen floor I fell and cut the underneath of my arm pretty bad and got some good bruises. It left me a little sore and then I had to clean the carpet in the living room and squirt him off in the shower. The moveable shower arm that our neighbors gave us has been the best thing ever. I think I will make an appointment to talk with someone this week and see about options. I think I won't go to church tomorrow and just stay home and play catch-up with myself. I've got so much to do and I seem worn out all the time. Susie came to visit tonight while Craig was with Steve, Wendy, the girls and Carl at the July 4th Spectacular. Craig was very excited to go with them. He loves being with the children and grandchildren. I would have got some of my work done, I think, but it was nice to visit with her. Craig ran the 4th of July 10K and only made it five miles before he just stopped running and became very disoriented. And, again he was at a slant and not knowing what was going on around him. It was very kind of Richard to take him and bring him home. I just had him rest most of the day and stay out of the sun. I think this will be his last race. He didn't even know that he hadn't finished.

July 6, 1998. *"Be the best of whatever you are"* — Today was Jamison's first birthday. Suzanne had the party at the park and had dinner. It was a great time. The children all played so cute together. Suzanne had a great dinner for everyone. I went over and got Taylor and Madison so Wendy could get her payroll done since Steve is still in North Carolina. It thrills me to see the children play together. They are all so cute and Craig loves to watch them. Jamison had a great time and looked so cute. Craig seemed to enjoy himself and the Clark's are kind to sit and chat with him. I am so exhausted tonight after crying so much yesterday and last night. There are not enough hours in the days.

July 7, 1998. *"He never said it would be easy, He only said it would be worth it"* — Craig volunteered today. He cried this morning. It was hard to take him today. Marsha, the owner of the Alzheimer's facility, visited me tonight when I picked Craig up. She wanted to know if I viewed him as declining over the past two months as much as they have. He's been going there for five months now. And, yes, he has declined the past two months. Sometimes he seems more coherent than others. Sometimes I almost convince myself that he's okay. I'm taking Friday off with Suzanne and going to Park City for her birthday. I've scheduled a massage for her and a nail appointment for me. We're going to go have a nice lunch and shop and have a wonderful day. Su is going to pick Craig up that day and take him to volunteer and hopefully he will spend the night and she will pick him up the next morning and bring him home. I feel excited and looking forward to something for the first time in a long time. Even when I went to New York I didn't feel excited because I knew I was leaving him with the children and it made me nervous. I know that I'm leaving him with caregivers that I am paying and that he's spending the night and I don't need to rush for anything. He literally does not know how to dress or undress at all anymore. I went to a grief support group with Su tonight. It was helpful in that the girl that directed it was the same one that talked about the stages of Alzheimer's one night at a care facility. She is going to have a social worker call me tomorrow and have someone visit Craig to evaluate him. It should be an interesting week after I talk to them and then talk to my doctor friend on Thursday. I'm educating myself more every day.

July 9, 1998. *"And let us not be weary in well doing: for in due season we shall reap, if we faint not"* (Galatians 5:9) — Suzanne's (our angel) 28th birthday. What joy she has brought into our life. Craig was so thrilled the night of her birth. He was truly a wonderful father that thought of his children as jewels. Oh, so much has happened in the last 28 years. Steve got back from North Carolina last night and called me this morning to say Hi. He is taking Taylor and Madison to Seven Peaks for the day. I'm taking the day off tomorrow to spend with Suzanne. Su will pick Craig up and take him to the Alzheimer's Center. He is going to spend the night but he doesn't know. He's very confused tonight and talking and making no sense. He's talking a lot about running races. He told me that I give him too many big pills and that's why his brain doesn't work. He had another accident today and it was everywhere. Suzanne washed the rugs and the clothes and Craig tried to clean up the bathroom himself. He just cried when I got home and said he was trying to do what I always do and it just didn't work. He said he wanted to be just like me. I just tried to hold him and laugh about why he or anyone else would want to be like me — that was a silly thought. I told him our house needed one of me and one of him and there was no other way so he needed to like himself because I do. I told him to get his clothes off and he could get in the tub. He can't undress himself anymore. I went to see a doctor today and we talked about medications and he gave me two "handicap" tags for the car. I gave Suzanne one so she could have one when she has her dad with her. You just need to take a paper signed by the doctor to Motor Vehicle Division and for no charge they give you two tags. Or, you can give them your car registration and license plate number, $5 and they will give you new plates with the handicapped sign. That seemed like something more than I needed. This will be wonderful when you have him with you. It is so hard to have him walk very far when you take him anywhere. My mind just seems to go and go and I don't know what I'm doing from day to day anymore. I just feel overwhelmed. He wants to know when it's church every fifteen minutes.

July 12, 1998. *"That which does not destroy us makes us stronger"* (This was one of Craig's favorite sayings) — Friday was a great day with Suzanne. We went to Park City, had lunch and went for a walk. We then went to the outlet stores and shopped. We were back home by 4:30. Su picked Craig up around 9:00 that morning and took him to volunteer. She stayed with him until around 11:30. She is such an angel. She picked him up the next morning around 10:00 and he wasn't even aware that he spent the night. He wanted to go run and was gone for about an hour when Suzanne got a call from the Alzheimer's lost program. He had fallen down and someone used his tag to call. He was very disoriented and didn't even know he had fallen. It took forever to get him into the car. He chipped a tooth, hit his head, and scraped his knee and his knee looks a little swollen as well. At least I know he won't want to run for a couple of days. We went to Collins' cabin and had a great evening. He enjoys being around them. We always laugh a lot when we are together. Jim's one son commented that Craig was too young to have 'Old Timers Disease' when they were told Craig had Alzheimer's. We got home late and went right to bed because Craig got up early to run with Richard and Bob this morning. He so wanted to go to church and visit with Mike. So I got him showered and dressed and a neighbor came down and stayed with him and then took him to Priesthood. I brought him home, changed his clothes and had him watch golf for a while so I could go to work and then I had him eat a sandwich. I've decided an easy one is a sandwich wrapped up in a flour tortilla and it all stays together and is easy to eat with little mess. We rested for a little and then went to Susie's and had a barbecue with Joan, Bonnie and Ernie. It was fun to visit with them and it's always good for people to see Craig's deterioration so they understand a little better.

July 13, 1998. *"Look for the oak tree in the acorn"* — Craig is beginning to question the pills I give him and say he doesn't need them. Then at bedtime after a bath he'll take his sleeping pills and not say anything. He got upset while he was in the tub and said he couldn't go to lunch with Jesse tomorrow because he wanted to go get his day over with. I'm almost beginning to think he's feeling comfortable out there as Suzanne said, "it's his world and he doesn't need to fit into our world." I've tried to just stare him down and laugh when he gets upset or swears. I keep telling him that isn't nice language and he tells me, "well you say that too" — and I said that I don't and he says, "Oh, you're not perfect all the time," and we laugh. He wanted to brush his teeth tonight and remembered how. He even turned his own water off and that's unusual. He couldn't remember how to put his underclothes on or how to put his slippers on and he told me not to look at his dinky because I wouldn't do anything anyway. He ate his ice cream tonight and spilled it on his jeans and his shorts because he doesn't know how to hold the bowl up, but he did eat it without sitting at the table. Hospice is going to call me tomorrow to evaluate him. They cover expenses for care if they think he has less than six months to live. I also have a social worker sending me information about Medicaid/Medicare to talk about finance options. What's sad is that they even ask if you have life insurance you can use. If you have a life insurance policy that has cash value you are expected to use it. You can remain the beneficiary but someone else needs to own the policy. I'm learning more as the end is getting closer. I hope I can help someone and change some health care legislation when this is all said and done.

July 14, 1998. *"I am only one, but I am one. I can't do everything, but I can do something and what I can do, I ought to do. And what I ought to do with the grace of God I will do"* — Craig spent the day at the Alzheimer's Center and is staying tonight. It seems nice and yet strange. I feel like we are in the middle of two worlds and not fitting into either one. Death could be sweet. Vista Hospice Care is visiting Craig tomorrow to evaluate him. Jesse will pick him up from the center for lunch and then bring him home. Steve called tonight and was shocked that his dad was spending the night there. We are still trying to play catch-up with the store. It is doing better. Suzanne and the children picked me up to go get a slurpee in the jeep with the top off. It was fun to go doing something fun and adventurous. I did get all the rugs and towels washed tonight. Craig got up in the night and urinated all over the bathroom. I've got three sets of rugs that I use. I almost feel guilty that he's there tonight when I'm home and I don't need to be anywhere. It feels good in a lot of ways but very strange to be alone even though I've been alone for at least two years now.

July 15, 1998. *"Whosoever will be great among you, let him be your minister, and whosoever will be chief among you, let him be your servant"* (Matthew 20:26-27) — Craig did well at staying all night. I tried to act like I went no where except work and we always take pills. Jesse picked him up and took him to lunch with Mel and Sandy. He said they had a good time. He then brought Craig home and turned the television on for him. I had Amber from Vista Hospice Care visit today and talk with Craig to evaluate him for aides in the morning and night. She said he qualified for hospice. I am very appreciative of the help and she will stop by my office tomorrow to have me fill out and sign the papers and have a doctor sign off. I told her ahead of time that Craig thinks he volunteers and that he won't get worse with the Alzheimer's. He talked non-stop with her and even started to cry when he talked about kidney problems and me having breast Cancer and almost dying. He said how lucky we are. I just put my arm around him, cried myself and wiped away his tears and tried to help him blow his nose, but he just snuffed and sniffled instead of blowing. I just listened and tried to fill in the blanks. I feel like I'm trying to stay one step ahead in seeking help as he slips further into the late stages of Alzheimer's. Our friends have been very supportive and some of them want to help but don't know how. I had a hard time getting him in the tub tonight and will be grateful for an aide to help me physically because tonight was very hard. I couldn't get his pants on without a struggle. I'll fill out the papers tomorrow to see if I can't receive help. They want bank statements for 36 months back, burial plans, cemetery certificates and even life insurance and its cash value along with safe deposit box contents. It's unbelievable that you are robbed of your mate and if you are able to get help financially, robbed of everything you have worked your whole life for. Su is going to stop by tomorrow and take him to volunteer and stay for the night again. We are going to go to Salt Lake and have dinner with an old school friend.

July 17, 1998. *"When ye are in the service of your fellow beings ye are only in the service of your God...and if I, whom ye call your king, do labor to serve you, then ought not ye to labor to serve one another?" (Mosiah 2:17-18)* — Su and I went to Salt Lake last night and had dinner. We visited until almost 10:00 and I came home feeling life is pretty good. I've decided that if you like yourself and have faith in yourself you can tough it out through most situations. We laughed most of the 50 miles home. She really laughed when I told her I had night blindness. We got lost going up and had some good laughs and going home even more laughs. I think we were both ready for a night away from reality. I dropped her off and then got lost in the trailer park and could not find my way out. I called her on my cell phone and we both laughed until our stomach's hurt. I don't know when I've felt so relaxed or not thought of anything. I came home, worked for an hour and went to bed and slept until almost 7:30. I was even able to get in the tub this morning. Craig was a little confused when I picked him up today, but he didn't realize that he spent the night again. I think I'll graduate to three nights per week next week and go Monday, Wednesday and Friday. I'm hoping I can have aides start this next week from Hospice.

They will come in the mornings and shave, shower and dress him. It will be wonderful to have their help. I almost feel like I'm part of the living world again. I've tried to stay upbeat and happy every day, but it's been wearing on some days and hard to keep everything in perspective. Suzanne had a good talk with her dad's sister this week. His family has not seen him since the first of June. She told her that we could no longer take Craig to their homes. If they want to see him they would have to come and see him. I appreciate her caring and concern. She is very honest and up front with everyone and not afraid to speak her mind. She deserves to be blessed beyond measure. She is blessed. I can't believe she turned 28 this month and that Steve will be 32 on Friday, July 24th. When the nurse came today to give him a physical checkup from Hospice he went to shake Craig's hand and Craig kept shaking my hand. Finally, I just said come on in Andrew we're glad to meet you. I told Craig he was from the clinic and in reality I didn't need to tell him anything because he kept asking if he was from one of the shoe manufacturers. I made eye contact and he said yes, I'm with that company. Craig now thinks that this shoe manufacturing company will pay us if we volunteer at the Alzheimer's Center. He asked Craig how much he weighed and I would just give him hand signals from behind Craig's head. When he asked how tall he was I said I thought 5'11" is a good height. When he asked Craig what day it was he told him number three. He didn't know if he was 8, 42 or 90. When he asked him who was President - he said president of what? And, when he said President of the United States, Craig thought and thought and then finally said, "I know he runs, he looks good, I don't like him, but I can't think of his name." I left him alone for an hour while I went back to work to get my brief case and turn off my computer and tie up loose ends. When I got home he had had an accident, trying to get it cleaned up from the toilet and crying. I cleaned up, told him everything was okay and then I got him to eat and get in the tub. He's asleep while he's watching television right now and I've somehow got to get him into bed. Steve just called back on his way to Big Rock Candy Mountain to tell his dad that he loved him. I told him he was in bed but that I would tell him first thing in the morning. Things seem to be moving rather rapidly now and it makes my heart flutter. Steve said he wanted to know that he is the person he is because of the training that he has had from us and he wants his dad to know how much he means to him and how much he is because of what he taught him. We all know it's coming. It's amazing that each day we can look at all this and laugh at the things Craig says and does. He was sad and upset when he went to bed tonight. I think he has hemorrhoids again.

July 19, 1998. *"When we serve, we gain more than we give"* — Craig went running early with his friends. He got confused because they went to Payson and it was different. He came home and got ready for church and went late with Mike and I didn't go at all. He came home and said that was the right amount of time. He's so innocent with his honesty that you want to chuckle but he wouldn't understand. He loves meat pies and that's what I had for him for lunch. We rode up to Salt Lake with Mike and Linda and had lunch and a lot of laughs. Craig was exhausted when we got home. He gets worn out easily. I left him with Suzanne to check on him and went with Collins for a sandwich. I was probably gone for two hours. When I got home Craig was close to tears because he had gone to the bathroom by himself and said he had to ask Heavenly Father to help him. I laughed with him and got him into the tub and then out for his nightly cup of hot chocolate, which I think, must soothe him. I need to talk to Steve and Suzanne tomorrow about their dad. We need to all pull together now and realize we are in this as one unit. I pray for the Lord to help each one of us to cling on for strength.

July 21, 1998. *"As for me and my house, we will serve the Lord."* (Joshua 24:15) — Yesterday Craig went with Jim, an old high school friend from Boston. They went to the cleaners and visited with Kent and walked around Harmon Park and some of the places they remembered as children growing up. He is here for the summer and enjoys spending time with Craig and reminiscing about the old days. It's wonderful to have friends like this. Craig said they walked a lot and talked a lot. Suzanne forgot until about 3:00 that she hadn't fed him lunch and knew that we were going to dinner with Rebecah and Cory at 5:00. They came out from Pennsylvania to visit Craig. Rebecca was one of Craig's employees. He adored her. Cory was great to sit back and listen as we reminisced. We had a great evening. We hope to see them one last time before they go back home to Pennsylvania. I am trying to cram all of the memories I can in for him while he has a flicker left. He is deserving of so much. He did not want to go volunteer today and when I told him he couldn't go with his mother he called me a liar. His mother was going to a home show and said he could come tomorrow. Suzanne said everyone needs a dose of reality in his decline. Perhaps it is more denial. I don't know. I've learned not to think about it and just do what I know I need to do each day for the two of us to survive.

July 24, 1998. *"Attitude – it's your choice"* — Steve's birthday and he is 32 today. I remember 32 years ago as though it were yesterday. Craig was so proud of becoming a father. He told the world. He was so happy. He was still playing baseball at the time of Steve's birth. He hit a grand slam, triple, double and single. It was an unbelievable game. Steve, Wendy and the girls are down at Big Rock Candy Mountain for the weekend. I had Craig volunteer yesterday and spend the night. Jim took him for the morning and visited with Trisha and Kent and had ice cream, then took him out to the Alzheimer's Center about 1:00. He has been wonderful to pick Craig up and visit all of his old stomping grounds as a youngster. It baffles him how Craig can recite stories of his youth and not know how to get in and out of the car or hold an ice cream cone. I had Alex and Emily over last night for a while and it took my mind off leaving Craig. It was nice to laugh and take a bubble bath. They called at 9:00 and told me that if Judy knew he was staying then he could sleep in his "own" bed in the "motel" part. I thought that was good news. I worked half day and then went shopping with Suzanne and the children. We then stopped and all picked Grandpa Craig up together. I thought it would be good for them to see where Grandpa volunteers. It made me feel good to bring him home. I guess it goes back to do unto others and I would want him to bring me home. He just chatters on and on and doesn't realize the other things that are going on around him. He was very excited to see us and said he did everything perfect when he was there and that he liked the food. He wanted to go back because he said he left money there. I try to always let him keep a few dollars in his pocket. I think he had a $5 bill. We told him we would get it next time we go volunteer. I had him get in a hot tub and take his pills. I'm hoping that I can get him to bed as soon as it gets dark. I want to go to bed early myself tonight. I've got to go get the car serviced tomorrow early and then I need to go to the Laundromat and wash all of Craig clothes and bedding.

July 25, 1998. *"Even sunshine burns if you get too much"* — Craig got up late since I didn't need to wake him up. I had an appointment to get the car serviced at 9:30 and it was dark and rainy. I fixed breakfast (his cereal in a huge bowl and the biggest spoon we have) and left him to eat while he talked to himself. He keeps saying keeping it square. I finally learned from Bill that is what he would say to Craig at the golf course – keep it square. It really sunk in. Everything is "keeping it square." I told him I would be back after he ate and he could just watch television. I got back one hour later and he was hunched over the breakfast table and had not moved since he finished eating his cereal. I watch him take his pills any more because he sometimes puts them in the glass or drops them, as he becomes more confused. I put him in the tub instead of the shower since I didn't need to be anywhere. He watched television in the bedroom while I did a little work. I worked at the store today for the last two hours of the day and cleaned it up and brought the entire old advertising posters home and just mucked out a little. I seem to have less ambition and drive and I'm tired a lot. I don't really feel depressed, but I think it is just the stress of everything. I could just lie around and that isn't like me at all. I got Craig fish and chips for lunch. He loves fish lately and it is something he can eat pretty well with his fingers by himself. I got him a yogurt tonight and he said it was the best thing he had ever eaten — even better than the fish. He couldn't sit on the couch and eat it though. He has to eat everything at the table and he tried to sip out of the spoon. I told him he had to pick the spoon up with his hand and eat it. It wasn't a drink with a straw. He didn't know the difference. Steve stopped by and visited for about an hour until we were on the third round of the same stories. I've heard them all so much that I can pretty well tell who or what he's talking about. He talked about an old BYU buddy that doesn't have a dinky anymore. He had some radical surgery done several years ago when he had Cancer and then he went on to talk about another friend that had the same surgery. He doesn't know a spoon from a straw or what you do with either, but he can remember something that happened many years ago. He doesn't know their names and you fill in the blanks. He was the one millionth fan at the Smith Fieldhouse for BYU basketball and he remembers that by saying he has the old basketball that McGee is going to shine up for him and he was too shy to get up to say anything and no one knows what he is talking about. He talks about Jesse taking him to lunch a lot. He is known at the Alzheimer's Center as the one that likes to talk to everyone a lot but of course he thinks he's 'volunteering' and helping. He definitely can talk a lot. It's no wonder his mouth gets dry and it's not just from the anti-depressants that he takes. He talks to himself all the time too now. I think if I could get him qualified for hospice, that would help with getting him to the center as well. I know that it is a labor of love to shave, shower, dress and feed him every morning; but labor also means it is wearing and hard. I've got to get him transitioned there if I'm going to go back to New York again to work for a week. There is no way that I could leave him in the care of Steve and Suzanne like I did before. He tells everyone that they have the blood and the medicine just perfect and so it's just like he doesn't have Alzheimer's any more. Pat called tonight to bolster my ego and tell me everything is okay. I love her dearly.

July 27, 1998. *"Believe"* — Yesterday I got Craig up to go run. I don't know, as I will do that anymore. It's becoming harder and harder to wake him up — let alone dress him. He came home and I got him ready for church and then let Mike pick him up for the last part of Sunday School. I went to Sacrament meeting by myself. I only put golf socks on Craig anymore because the crew socks are too hard to pull on his feet. He's like dead weight and doesn't know how to pick his feet up or anything. The only time I put a belt on him is on Sunday's because he can hardly pull down his own pants let alone handle a belt. I noticed as we were walking out of the house in the afternoon that he had wet his pants. I told him he had sat in some water and we needed to change his pants. I finally got them changed without him taking off his shoes and then we went in circles for at least one minute while I tried to button his pants. I finally was laughing so hard from the circles that I held him still and had him try to button them himself. He got them buttoned and then I zipped them. We went to Mike and Linda's for a barbecue and when we are out and away from home I am reminded more and more of how hard it is for him to feed himself, sit and just do simple things for himself. He did not want to go volunteer today and he stayed home with Suzanne and the children. They went running a few errands and Craig got tired and had a little nap. Rebecca and her husband, Cory stopped by to see him before they left to go back to Pennsylvania. When I came home at the end of the day he was sitting on the toilet and crying his eyes out. It took me 30 minutes to calm him down and have him eat and get in the tub. I gave him an anti-depressant pill and a sleeping pill with his dinner. I shampooed his hair and let him soak for about 15 minutes and then got him out and let him watch Larry King. He likes that and we had a cup of hot chocolate and shared a doughnut. I told him it didn't have any sugar since he thinks he can't eat sugar anymore for some reason. He loved his dinner that Suzanne fixed—stir-fry chicken with rice. He ate a lot and I kept wiping away his tears and giving him kisses to soothe him. I still don't know what it was all about. He did say he wanted to jump off a cliff but he wouldn't do that. My heart aches for him.

July 29, 1998. *"Drop a word of cheer and kindness, just a flash and it's gone, but there's half-a-hundred ripples circling on and on and on"* — I picked Craig up at 4:00 today from "volunteering" and he was a little angry with me. He said he stayed two days and where have I been. I told him I was just to work and he wasn't there for two days. He was very agitated and I gave him an anti-depressant before we got to Camille's to get his hair cut. We had dinner and I got him in the tub early. He had a bowel movement in the tub again. He has his pills down him and I'm hoping I can get him to bed early. Suzanne and the children came over for a little bit to visit. Craig's brother, Cary, has stopped by to visit the last two days with Craig and we haven't been home. I guess having Steve try to call him 2-3 times has helped. I hope he stops by tomorrow. Cary hasn't seen Craig since last summer. He'll be shocked by his deterioration. Jesse called as well. He has been a great friend. I'm trying to figure out how I'm going to go to New York next week. I hope if Suzanne, Steve, Jesse and perhaps Cary visit or take him to lunch it won't be so bad. I'm hoping. I somehow need to approach him on Saturday and give him a calendar as to how many days I will be gone and then pick him up. He can mark off the days somewhat like a little child leaving his parent(s). Actually, I don't think he understands time – days. I've got to get him some more shorts and socks. He actually fed himself pretty well tonight and he said he liked the food they had at the center. I've got to call his friends tonight and get next week scheduled out. It's all closing in. Steve called tonight on his way to Salt Lake to visit with the Utah Homeowners Association. Basically life is pretty good. If only we could all realize how fragile life is and live our lives as such at a very early age and live accordingly. I wouldn't want to go backwards but I wish I knew ten years ago what I know today and I would handle some things differently, especially money and insurance matters. Tricia called to encourage me along and check on Craig. I feel so blessed to have such friends.

August 2, 1998. *"I am sending an angel ahead of you to guard you along the way to bring you to the place I have prepared" (Exodus 23:20)* — I'm alone tonight and Craig is staying at the Alzheimer Center. I'm sure he's angry with me tonight. Yesterday we went to visit Steve/Wendy and the girls. On the way home I mentioned about staying overnight if I went to a meeting and he became very upset. I was even a little frightened. I gave him an extra sleeping pill last night before he went to bed and I got up and went to church by myself and let him sleep. I got him up and we had pot pies for lunch with Su and a lot of laughs talking about old school friends and filling in the blanks. I said I was going to run to work for a while and Su asked Craig to go to the post office with her and that she was then going to go volunteer for a while and would he go with her. She said he got very nervous and anxious. I'm sure when the staff told him he did not like me very well. I'm sure he feels betrayed and that I'm the enemy. I can handle that as long as the children know that this is a good thing and something that's needed. Suzanne and the children will visit him tomorrow and have lunch. Steve and Wendy said they would go out as well. I'll call Jesse in the morning and see if he will go out for lunch one day. Su is leaving Wednesday to go back to Nevada City. I think I'm going to be lost without her support and understanding of being a caregiver. I'm leaving for New York for a week to work so next weekend I'll fill in the blanks hopefully of the week at the Center and a week away for me.

August 8, 1998. *"For He will command His angels concerning you to guard you in all your ways" (Psalms 91:11)* — I brought Craig home this morning from the Alzheimer's Center where he stayed for a week while I went to New York. Marsha, from the center, was so kind to leave me voice messages at night and tell me how he was doing. Suzanne took him 2-3 times and Jesse and Jim each took him to lunch. Steve and Carl picked him up and took him to Strawberry to look at Carl's Cabin to fix up.

Steve took him to their home. He had dinner with Steve, Wendy and the girls. He took him back to the Center. Steve is still struggling with this disease and all of the every day things that go along with it. It breaks his heart to see his dad's deterioration and decline like a baby requiring so much assistance. He's a lot better about wearing diapers. We went to Collins' cabin tonight for dinner. They have been so kind. They are like family. I'm so very appreciative of their kindness. They adore our children and how they help their dad. We are indeed very blessed.

When Suzanne went out to get him the first time she went up to the gate and didn't have a key or the combination. I forgot to tell her there was a button you could push to activate the gate. All the residents walking around just smiled and waved and they didn't know what she was doing or saying. I laughed my head off when she was telling me. She finally had Alex climb the fence and go get Grandpa. He did. Craig came out, said, "Hi" got a drink out of the fountain and just stood there. Alex had to go back in and get one of the aides to help get them in and Grandpa out. I just pictured it and laughed. She said he was pretty good about wearing diapers all week long. I thought he would be upset when I picked him up but he gave me a hug and seemed content to be there. That makes me feel better about having him there.

August 9, 1998. *"Keep on loving each other... for by so doing some people have entertained angels without knowing it" (Hebrews 13:1,2)* — I let Craig sleep in a little and I had a diaper on him and he was dripping wet when I got him up. We showered before eating breakfast. I had to change all of the bedding. It's hard to believe that everything could be so wet. He looks so bewildered. I tell him he's sweaty because he got hot. He believes me and/or doesn't know the difference. He watched television most of the day. He went to part of church with Mike and I had a diaper on him to go today. He doesn't mind it as bad as I thought. Tonight when I got him out of the tub he cried and didn't want it and then relented and said okay. It is quite an experience putting a diaper on an adult the first time. He would stand still and I would stand behind him and hold it in place with my knee while I brought it up and around to hook the front. I then would put a pair of jockey shorts over it to hold in place. He had an accident before I put him into the tub tonight and it really upset him.

When I put him to bed tonight he just cried and called himself dumb and was I going to put him in jail. I don't know what that one meant. One of his friends called tonight to inquire about him and said he was too busy to stop by. I believe people are still in denial or else they just can't handle seeing someone their own age with a disease like Alzheimer's. One of his friend's said he was giving me a $100 a month to help care for Craig. Life is definitely about caring and doing for others. We went to Collins' cabin and ate dinner with them. They have been wonderful to Craig.

August 10, 1998. *"One of the wonderful things of life is a sense of belonging"* — The start of another week. Craig volunteered again today. He wasn't excited about it but I told him that Suzanne was sick. (She had a Migraine headache). Jim picked him up again today and took him roaming around the city. Craig keeps losing his sunglasses when he is with him. I only buy the very cheap variety anymore. It was a hectic day. We stopped to get something to eat on the way home (to eat at home). He didn't like the pizza I got very well. It's limiting to buy or prepare food for him that is easy for him to eat as finger-food. I got him in the bathtub after he had another accident. When he sits on the toilet - he doesn't realize that he is having a bowel movement and it is all over the back of the toilet seat and his butt and so it takes quite a bit of wiping to get he and the toilet cleaned. It upsets him and he thinks he's dumb. I put a diaper on him tonight and he just cried again. I held him and told him how much I loved him; it hurt me to see him cry and that I was just trying to help him. I don't know what he started to think about but he said he understood and it was just about getting square and then everything is okay. (I believe he's talking about getting squared up to swing a golf club and he is just confusing things). This is an ugly disease. Jack told me that he was listening to a report where they are doing studies about Alzheimer's being caused by some type of bacteria. I'm glad that they are searching all avenues. From everything I read and understand it will be at least another ten years before there is anything that is going to slow or alter the process of this disease.

August 11, 1998. *"Hold onto love and loyalty"* — Another day of volunteering. Last night was hard in that he didn't want to wear the diaper and said he would be smart. We both cried. Tonight he said right up front that he would wear one. He's frightened of using the bathroom anymore. We had a power outage this morning and so I had to go buy a flashlight, checkout the fuse box and then call an electrician because we had no power to the bathroom and the one middle bedroom where Craig watches television. I panicked until I could get an electrician here because Craig is frightened of the dark and I needed to get him into the bathroom and the tub to get him washed off. He went willingly to volunteer today knowing that Suzanne was sick. He'll do anything if it will help his children. Tonight when I picked him up they had been dancing. I believe he is feeling more comfortable out there.

August 12, 1998. *We are each of infinite worth and have a divine & individual mission"* — Another hard day. I took Craig to the doctor this morning to have him see Craig and have him "hopefully" sign the papers so we could have hospice. He didn't sign the papers and said he wanted Craig to have a spinal tap to make sure there is no swelling on the spine and eliminates everything — like we haven't run every imaginable test to eliminate everything. I wanted to ask him who would pay for this and how we could get Craig to understand and what would happen if anything went wrong and left him paralyzed. I really wanted to say live with and take care of him for 24 hours and then say he isn't into the late stages of Alzheimer's and should not qualify for hospice. He said he didn't want me to get my hopes up. I assured him that I was far above getting my hopes up after all these years. And, when he asked me about living wills, etc. I wanted to say, "give me a break". I cried all the way home knowing that once again he was not going to receive Hospice. I can't believe some of the healthcare professionals. I called IHC and requested another primary care physician for him. Craig stayed home with Suzanne this afternoon while I ran between doctors. He had a few accidents while I was away. It was hard for her today as well. She also is realizing that we are all getting "there" and it is a hard pill to swallow. He still knows us. He just can't do anything for himself or help us help him. Heartbreaking for everyone.

August 13, 1998. *"Live in the present – life is for the living"* — What a day. We started off with the toilet flooding and me not knowing it until there was an inch of water. We had an 11:15 doctor appointment with the

Alzheimer's Pharmacology Research study with no time to spare. I had to shave Craig, squirt him off in the shower and get him dressed. I had cried a lot the night before thinking that a physician that knows nothing about being a caregiver or anything about Alzheimer's tells me not to get my hopes up, but he thinks Craig should have a spinal tap to eliminate a disease I know he doesn't have. The disease he is talking about with pressure on the spine he would have had bowel problems early on and he is just become incontinent in the past two months. We needed to take a urine sample with us because he couldn't "pee in the cup" last time — he called it "peeing in the pail". I tried to pull down the diaper and have him urinate in the bottle. He would keep saying "pee-pee-pee-pee" trying with all his might like a little kid and then saying, "pee in the pail - pee in the pail - pee in the pail". I would pull the diaper and pants up try to get myself ready and assure him it was okay, and he would just keep saying "pee - pee - pee - I can do it". Finally, after 30 minutes he started to "pee" and he was so excited that he could do it - pee in the pail. I was so distraught from the morning and the day before. I called my doctor friend who helped me through this so Craig could get signed off for Hospice. He called a neurologist and he called me back in five minutes. He wants me to bring Craig with me on Monday and he requested another MRI so we went to Salt Lake to the pharmacology research place, back home to "volunteer." They called at 3:30 and said they had an appointment at 5:30. I had to hurry and leave, go get a prescription of Valium to calm him down for an MRI (in the past he's claustrophobic – perhaps he's not any longer) and then go to the Alzheimer's center, get him, and get him to the hospital for the MRI. We got there and they had an emergency and so we had to wait for an extra hour. I didn't get him dressed before we went home. He could hardly eat tonight.

August 14, 1998. *"Stress is manageable"* — Today was the worst yet. Craig was the most confused as I have ever seen him. He ate some cereal after I got him showered. He was so wet (sweaty as I tell him) when he got up even with the diaper that we showered before breakfast. He kept going on and on about me lying to him and I believe it was yesterday when I tried to get a urine sample and he had a hard time being able to urinate on cue. He was harder to dress and a lot more confused about how to get in and out of the car and into the Alzheimer's Center today.

I'm having him stay the weekend. Richard and Bob will pick him up on Sunday and bring him home in the afternoon. They are such good friends. Last week Craig told one of his friends that he was forty years old and had not had sex in fifty years. The friend laughed about that one. Craig put his sock on his hand and didn't know that it wasn't his foot. Last night before he went to bed he said he wanted a chocolate from the cupboard where I keep a box of chocolates. He was so lucid - walked to the cupboard and took the box of chocolates and then dropped all but one on the floor. I picked up the chocolates, threw them in the garbage, and handed him the one chocolate left and he said, "I want you to have it." I tucked him in bed and cried. This was my Craig. He was always so generous and kind.

August 15, 1998. *"Make order out of chaos"* — It was a difficult day. I woke up knowing I was alone and could be leisurely about getting ready for our neighbor's funeral. It made me more aware of things I need to think about. Cary called this morning and wanted the address of the Alzheimer's Center to visit Craig and take some pictures. I hope that he did. Bob and Richard will pick him up tomorrow afternoon and bring him home. I sometimes wish he could fall asleep and not wake up so I wouldn't have to have him in a Center to live, and some days I think he can stay home with me forever with help, but after Friday I don't think that any more. I need to study more about what is ahead and start preparing for the inevitable. I don't know what we would do without family and friends that love and care about us. I was so tired last night after I got home that I crawled into bed with no sheets or pillowcases. I threw a comforter over me and slept through the night until almost 7:30. I've been scatterbrained these past few days and am having a harder time concentrating on the things I need to do day-to-day. I just sit and stare into space when I'm home alone. I don't even care if I go anywhere to be around people.

August 16, 1998. *"Have the courage to be imperfect while striving for perfection"* — I slept through the night after a long bubble bath in the dark. I got up this morning, sat and watched the Today show before getting ready for church. It was Liz's homecoming. It was a great meeting. I came home and went to brunch with Pat & Tricia. We had omelets and orange juice that tasted so good. I felt spoiled. We then went to some shops and walked around. It was nice, but I always feel like I need to hurry home for Craig. Richard and Bob picked him up at 4:30, brought him home and sat and visited for about an hour. They are truly great friends. We walked up the street together to say "welcome back" to Liz. They sent us home with food for Craig's dinner. He had on a wet/messy diaper and I let him finish eating before we got in the tub. He struggled to know how to eat the sandwich and chips. I let him soak in the tub for a long time tonight after I scrubbed him down and washed his hair. He wanted hot chocolate and fell asleep watching TV and questioned me when I said the news was over, it's 10:00 and time to go to bed. He did better in the dark tonight, but went to the wrong bedroom. It took me a minute to get him to the right bed.

August 19, 1998. *"Stressed spelled backward spells desserts"* — Craig went with me to the neurologist today. He told us the results of the MRI. There is more atrophy at the frontal part of the brain compared to the atrophy on the sides two years ago. He had him walk with one foot in front of the other and he couldn't do it well but he did get his feet from side to side and he had him run down the hall and back. He did that pretty well and Craig reminded him that he was a marathon runner (he knew). He asked him how old he was and Craig said 12 plus one. Two years ago when they gave him verbal tests they had him add 12 plus one; so, I don't know if he retained that or not. He asked him what year it was and he said 1013. His birthday is the tenth month and the thirteenth day. Again, I don't know anymore what to think of his answers. He asked him who the prophet of his church was and he said Heavenly Father. He got my name right but gave his grandchildren's names instead of his children. He is in diapers 24 hours a day now. I had him stay at the center last night and picked him up tonight. He bumped his head twice getting into the car. One of the reasons I may decide to make his stay permanent is that I can't get him in and out of the car and I can hardly dress him by myself anymore. He doesn't understand how to lift his feet to help me and he is like deadweight. The hard part is that he still knows us. I have to cross the bridge that this is where I live and that he will live there and I go visit. The thought makes me sick inside, but I also know I can't do this much longer. It's hard to imagine that you don't know how to sit and then get your legs in the car. You panic wondering how you are going to get him from point A to B. Tonight I gave him a taco salad in a huge bowl and he kept eating it with his hands instead of a fork. Finger foods work the best. This is a horrible disease. I hope I can get Hospice to make it work so that others will know that it can be done. I plan to lobby the legislature so that laws regarding Alzheimer's can and will be changed.

August 22, 1998. *"Find inner harmony and peace"* — I picked Craig up today. He has been volunteering since Thursday morning. He thought I went to New York again. I can't dress or undress him. I'm struggling more now than I thought I would. It's hard to have to ask for help when you've been independent your whole life. Steve and Wendy said they would help me financially as well as some of his friends. I just feel overwhelmed by everything right now. I feel like I'm drowning. Suzanne said I'm depressed and I guess that is a fair estimate of where I am at right now because I'm having a hard time staying focused and doing the things I should be doing.

August 24, 1998. *"There is a time and season for all things"* — I feel good about myself tonight and yet I can't quit crying. I took Craig back to volunteer permanently yesterday after picking him up on Saturday. I got him up Sunday morning and the bed looked like someone had thrown chocolate milk shakes all over it and Craig head to toe. I can't even imagine now as I look back. I almost wanted to laugh instead of cry and I think if I would have had a camera I would have taken a picture. I do have a camera. I just have not had my wits about me for a long time. I felt focused and energized at work and want to get organized. I feel like the choices I made are right and that what I am doing now is the best for all of us, including Craig, because the time will be quality time. He needs more than one person to help him at a time and I couldn't be more than one person and I've never been able to have a doctor sign off on Hospice. Unbelievable. I love him dearly and I wish he could shut his eyes and have his time on this earth finished and he could return home to his Heavenly Father. He has led an exemplary life. They said he was agitated and upset last night when I left. I wished I would have let someone else take him out and yet for some strange reason I felt it needed to be me. They said he actually ran around the building by the fence and he hasn't run in a long time. They gave him two Nortriptolene tablets. I inquired about meds and Marsha said they would probably taper him off them after he's been out there for a while and transitions in. I think I will have Suzanne visit and take some more clothes and meds out, but not for a few days. I think she is struggling with my decision right now too because her dad still knows her and the children. I always thought that when this time came for full time care he wouldn't know us anymore. He does and it made the decision and the doing even harder. When I stopped by Steve and Wendy's to tell them what I did I could not stop crying. Steve put his arms around me and asked why I was crying. He reminded me that it was me that would constantly remind them how blessed we were that we had this wonderful person in our lives for as long as we did and that not many people are able to have the opportunity to say their good-byes to a loved one like we were able to with Craig during a two-year period of time. This is a crazy disease. In spite of it I feel incredibly blessed. A richer and a better person because of this experience with Craig and 'Big Al'. I need to give myself some healing time as well and spend time with family/friends and laugh again. Pat and Tricia both called me tonight to reinforce my decision and tell me it was the right thing to do. I love them dearly.

August 25, 1998. *Slogan on a clipper ship: "One hand for yourself and one hand for the ship" If you used both hands to scrub the ship, you would wind up in the water with the sharks. If, however, you hung on with both hands, you would get nothing done. To scrub the deck, you must learn to use one hand to take care of yourself while the other hand gets the job done." (This same formula applies to Caregivers)* — My third night alone. I've got a splitting headache tonight - it's 8:00 and I'm exhausted and ready for bed. I finally feel like I'm catching up at work. That is a good feeling. One of Craig's friends called tonight and wanted to visit him, a friend that hasn't seen him much in the past two years. He wanted to know how Craig's family has handled this. I feel sorry for them, too. The majority of people are in denial. I think I have truly become a more loving and caring person and learned more in the past two years than I have in a lifetime. I need to figure out how to approach the visits with Craig. I just want to put my arms around him, hold him and tell him that I love and care about him. I visited a new doctor today and he said he would be Craig's primary care physician. So, there is hope for Hospice. I feel like I've been constantly jumping through hurdles this past while trying to get things that I need to get through this. I don't know what we would be doing without our children and friends.

August 26, 1998. *"Rely on others for help and comfort not just yourself"* — I talked to Marsha at the Center today. Craig is known as the chatterbox and it makes me smile. Craig was always so quiet, shy and soft-spoken. He keeps asking where Judy is, and says he was only supposed to spend a half. I feel like I deserted him and would love to put my arms around him and just hold him and tell him how much I love him. I took some more clothes, meds and frozen foods and met her at the bank and gave them to her. I think it will be better if I don't visit for a week until he knows that is his home now. Suzanne is struggling right now too. She's tended her dad for two years, her first child goes to school all day, Emily has been sick and she got her second paps smear back as abnormal. I know how she feels. She knows we made the right decision, but it doesn't make it any easier to swallow. Craig's sister called her. Suzanne is the middle person and the psychiatrist for everyone. People must find it easier to talk to Suzanne than me about Craig. I, too, am very honest and upfront. I hold nothing back about his decline. I want the world to know about this wicked disease so that we can receive help. We need research. Steve called me this morning to let me know he is there to help me in whatever I need to do. My friend, Javan, sent me flowers today. People are very kind. Dave called yesterday and wants to go visit Craig. Marsha said that Craig ran outside in the sprinklers yesterday and the day before he ran around the fence. I'm sure he's befuddled by what's going on. My heart aches and I wish this could all go away. I wish we could all shut our eyes and this could be something that was a show we watched on television or a dream and we'll wake up soon.

September 5, 1998. *"Our understanding of life can be increased and made richer through friendships"* — It's been two weeks and I feel like I've deserted a friend by not writing. I've been back trying to jump through the hoops getting some of Craig's life insurance to help financially. You need three doctor's signatures stating that he has 12 months or less to live and fill out a report. Then we get that back and they want to see the doctor's records. I can see showing them the Power of Attorney and Legal Guardianship papers, but this other is ridiculous when it is your own money. I may end up borrowing rather than asking for some of it. The care at the Center went up $350 a month as well. My heart is touched with the kindness and love of his friends and their willingness to help. I volunteer on the weekends there. It makes me happy to be there with Craig. Last Saturday I curled the women's hair and shaved the men and gave them all hand massages and clipped or painted their nails. This Saturday I took hair clippers and gave Craig and all of the gentlemen a hair cut and shaved their necks. I love being there with Craig and helping. I've noticed that one resident is wearing his other pair of running shoes that I took out for him. That makes me feel good that the aides are comfortable with us that we want to share with the other residents. One of the patients fell down and cut her lip and then fell again and cut it worse. I helped them take her to her bed and waited for her nurse to come and give her a shot of Valium to calm her down. I need to re-read, because I think she has another disease and not Alzheimer's and perhaps redirecting medication - she could be a lot calmer. I helped care for Kurt yesterday and prepared him to graduate before his daughter came. I stayed with her and he died at 10:08 p.m. so peacefully that we both smiled as we cried. Death is sweet and we only administered three doses of morphine over a three-hour period. I had clipped his mustache, nails and dry skin from his lips and swabbed his mouth. When he died he didn't look parched any more. I'm sure his daughter is at peace today knowing her father is gone to be with her mother- his wife. She died of Cancer four years ago. I will be attending his funeral on Friday even though yesterday was my only full day caring for him or meeting his daughter. We shared a lot last night in celebrating his death. And, I was so impressed with the mortuary and the young gentleman that picked him up. It was wonderful and peaceful. They treat the body with so much respect and it is like an art in wrapping them up before putting them on the gurney and wheeling them away for one of their final rides. I'm very appreciative to the Center and Kurt's daughter that they allowed me to help with Kurt because I'm sure it helped prepare me for what is ahead with Craig. And, you can't have enough hands at an Alzheimer's home.

September 11, 1998. *"Ye cannot behold with your natural eyes, for the present time, the design of your God concerning those things which shall come hereafter, and the glory which shall follow after much tribulation. For after much tribulation come the blessings." (D&C 58:3-4)* — Today was Kurt's funeral. A wonderful tribute and I'm sure his children were thrilled with the accolades given to their father. Marcia from the Alzheimer's Center spoke. She is an angel. All of the aides are so dedicated. They are truly special people. I've decided I need to get them shirts that says Alzheimer's Center and we should all be proud to wear them. I liked the simplicity of the sunflowers and simple wild flowers they had for his casket instead of a large casket spray. I saw the mortician, a close friend, and told him I wanted to look at caskets because I want something very simple for Craig and nothing fancy. I would love for the children to sing "There's an Angel Amongst Us" — Perhaps they can learn the words and sing it on a tape and then we could play the tape as well as have them sing. Craig yesterday told Marsha that he shouldn't be there - he needed to be on the other side. She said it was like he knew where he should be or wanted to be. She is a very religious person and believes that this is part of her ministry. I love her outlook that we can all help and she's not afraid to tell me when she needs something that I can do. She is a remarkable lady. Wendy and the girls picked him up yesterday and we all had dinner at their house. We had a good time. Carl stopped by and took him back. We are all still struggling with the fact that he is there full-time. I know that I feel so good when I can spend the day there. He tells me he loves me and gives me a hug. Bill is going to visit tomorrow while I'm there. I'm excited when Craig's friends go to visit.

September 15, 1998. *"The fruit of the Spirit is love, joy, peace, long-suffering, gentleness, goodness, faith, meekness and temperance." (Galatians 5:22-23)* — It's late and I'm sitting here in the dark watching television. I find it hard to be at home at night. The silence and loneliness seem to overcome me. I miss Craig and being able to take care of him and have him sit by me until it is time to go to bed. I miss him terribly. I had become used to taking care of him. I look forward to the weekends and being able to spend the whole day there. I love being around him and the other residents. It makes me feel good to be there. Craig is good to help people there. He still looks so good. He walks more with a slant and is becoming unsure of his footing. Mike and Linda went to see him on Sunday. I took ice cream and cookies out for a treat before bed to spend a little time with him. I'll get the menus done by tomorrow night and go visit. (I volunteered to type up the menus for a five-week period of time so a registered dietician can sign off on them and they can be posted.) I also want to get some short socks for them. They have got to be easier to put on them than the crew socks. We gave them pedicures Saturday and putting their socks back on was a trial. I've decided that you can't have enough socks — especially with 20 people. I need to get ready for the Alzheimer's run and get some donations to them. I was feeling caught up and now I feel like I'm behind again. I need to call the race team about running and let the clinic know that I have to concentrate on taking care of Craig now and handle that additional cost and since a few of his friends have been so good to help me with the cost of his care that I don't want to ask for donations this year. Last year was the First Annual Alzheimer's Fun Run. Craig ran with the team last year and they awarded him a plaque because we gathered the most donations. I worked at the store and let the team members take him up. I wished I would have been there to see him accept the plaque. He said that because of them he would be able to live and see his grandchildren. He thinks he's still taking two white pills that will help him live forever like I told him in the beginning. He was so proud when he came home with the plaque. He told me that it belonged to me because I was the one that 'gathered' all the money – not him.

September 21, 1998. *"Cultivate a happy and loving heart"* — I had a great time visiting Craig on Saturday and again on Sunday. Mike and Linda visited him on Sunday and he told them that he hadn't seen me in a long time — he does not know time distinction at all anymore. He's also talking more and more about his interaction with the other residents. He talks about the things that Heavenly Father wants him to do before he goes to the other side and then he'll talk about something off the wall. He constantly chatters. For somebody that has always been quiet and shy it catches you off guard. Sunday they had someone else's pants on him and socks that didn't match. The pants were too short and I changed his clothing before I took him to Steve's to visit. Suzanne had one of Craig's friend's call today and say that there is no way he can make himself go out to see Craig in those surroundings. I wish this process wasn't so hard.

It is hard and lonely at night. I guess that is the time when I would spend the most time taking care of Craig.

September 22, 1998. *"So much of what is great has sprung from the closeness of family ties"* — Another night...this is the first night I have come home and stayed and been able to stay here. I cried when I talked to Craig's friend, Jesse. It makes me feel at peace with myself that I did what I had too in that Craig seems to be comfortable and at peace where he is. This is a nightmare disease and one that you feel like you are in life alone and swimming upstream. I have lived a lifetime in these past two years. I love Craig so much and know that we will be together in eternity. I look forward to that.

September 24, 1998. *"Somehow experience the joy of your journey"* — I went to visit Craig tonight and helped him with dinner. I cut his chicken and gave him a bite. I said, 'isn't the food wonderful here' (it is) and he said, 'no, it tastes like shit'. I cut another piece of chicken and he said, 'this is the best steak I ever ate.' You never know what's coming out of his mouth. I shaved him while I was there. He's wearing his Adidas shirt and had slacks on. He looked like handsome Craig. Suzanne went out and said she had to fight back the tears because he looked like her "dad" again until he started to talk. He's not as talkative as he has been in the past. He seemed more docile to me tonight and he wanted one of the aides to take him to the bathroom. He told me about one of the aides being his favorite. I left him visiting Suzanne and I took the children home with me. Alex in particular has a hard time seeing his grandpa out there. Kathy wants to have a fundraiser for Craig to raise awareness about the disease and help with money to care for Craig. Steve also talked about having a golf fundraiser. Perhaps in the spring.

October 11, 1998. *"Awaken each day with a purpose – add value to life"* — Craig had another psychological evaluation today. The BYU Comprehensive Clinic called and asked if they could have a graduate student test Craig. I thought it would be an interesting follow-up and agreed. Craig thought he was an old friend and starting talking about Big Al. The fellow I'm sure chuckled when he found out Big Al was Alzheimer's and that was the reason he was there talking to him. He learned early into the conversation that even though Craig had verbal skills he was unable to remain focused to answer any questions. I'm sure he would start a story and then go into some other story. And also unable to perform any of the tasks since he was unable to in August of 1996. In fact, his IQ was 62 when they tested him then. What was ironic is that the examiner knew nothing about Craig and a professor told me he described him as a distinguished, tall, and handsome looking man with a friendly smile and he named him 'Sam Snead' – a golfer. When you are testing someone like that you aren't able to use his or her real name. Craig would have been delighted with the nickname and the description. One of the aides told me that Craig did tell him he was 'volunteering' there and he could stay and volunteer as well. I'm sure he declined the offer.

October 13, 1999. *"Believe in yourself"* — Craig's 55th birthday. The children had a birthday party for him. I had a hard time at first with the idea but I am so glad we did. Suzanne sent out invitations to a few friends and we had it at Steve and Wendy's. He struggled with food and sitting, but it was so worth it. He thoroughly enjoyed every minute. He just smiled and it was wonderful. Some cried as they saw him and I know it was easier for them in these surroundings than at the Alzheimer's Center. They were all great around him. He actually appeared connected to some. I don't think he would have called them by name but he definitely recognized people and got so excited. He would start off on a story about some that were pretty accurate. I'm very appreciative of our children and that they took the initiative to make this happen. They also know that this will probably be the last. It was a very special day – a hard day – but a wonderful day to see Craig smile and happy and somewhat coherent. I took him back and when we pulled into the parking lot he asked what we were doing. I had to swallow hard and not cry. I know he was confused at being away. We went in and he told the aides about "the world being there" to his party. I helped get him ready for bed and tucked him in and said my good-byes. I cried all the way home. He is my very best friend – my soul mate – the love of my life.

October 25. 1998. *"Everyone pays their dues; everyone has problems/ struggles – no one is immune"* — I went to church today with Steve and Wendy to watch Madison and Taylor in a Primary program. They were so cute.

Craig would have been so proud. He loved to go watch the children 'perform' as he called it. I'm hoping that I've written and put it on a disk. I've think I've had a little depression lately. Work has been chaotic and I've had a harder time accepting the fact that Craig is no longer coming home at all or ever. Craig is content at the Alzheimer's Center. He was so thrilled that night that he kept saying he was embarrassed because the whole world was there. He seemed so happy. Bill visited him and brought him an apple to eat. He always brings fruit with him and helps Craig eat it. He has been a wonderful friend to Craig. When I went to volunteer on Saturday they said they had seen him spiral that week and they literally had to feed him. They covered him with an apron and when the apron was on he thought he was tied to the chair. They had to tell him he could get up. He can still talk but his skills are going down. He didn't know how to cross a threshold of a door and we went to sit in the swing outside and he didn't know how to sit back and swing and yet he could talk about his grandma and grandpa (deceased) and that they loved us. He would constantly repeat that his grandma loved me and his mother didn't. I kept telling him that his mother loved everyone. It is really true that how we treat others and what we do for others is what goes with us. I feel so honored to have been Craig's other "half" — and that his friends are my friends. I care for them and the way that they love Craig. They felt honored to be able to say Happy Birthday and Good-bye to him in surroundings that they all felt comfortable in. The children were insightful to have done that. It was good for our grandchildren too.

November 1, 1999. *"Each loving experience and relationship will enhance and enrich our lives"* — Life at the center is like a full moon is out. One resident said she was late for the cemetery and where were the keys, another needed a coat and hat so he could go cruise and he needed the keys to the third car on the left. Another said not to give any more milk out because she couldn't afford it. We told her that it was not hers and that they had put hers away and that they were using their own milk. They tell people to come and eat because they have paid for it already or that it is a church social. It is unbelievable the things they can say and do to make them believe. And with Craig I never knew what was going to come out of his mouth anymore. You just have to love them and talk and listen to them like everything is wonderful and fine. What a mission to be sent on. I learned from a fireside about Bro. Matthew Cowley that in order to be a good missionary you need to love your mission and all the people and companions in it. I truly love all of my companions and all the people at the Center that are in my mission. I love Craig and all that he has taught me and continues to teach me. He loves his children and grandchildren and he loved seeing Steve's deer. (I remember a story about Craig and Steve going hunting together. Steve came home and said do you know that dad doesn't take bullets for his gun – why does he even go with me? I told him he went with him because he loves being with you and treading those hills that you two love.) He loves going for rides with Suzie and getting lunch. LeRoy is going to go with her one of these next Fridays. I'm so appreciative. I've learned that if the eyes had no tears, the heart would have no rainbows. I cry each night I leave the Center and drive home by myself.

November 16, 1998. *"It is only with the heart that one can see"* — It has been a long time since I have written. It seems as though I come home and stare off into space. I truly believe it gets harder instead of easier. I believe that Craig knows that I am someone familiar but not who I am — in that I am his wife, Judy. He will recognize me as someone familiar because I visit daily and he will say, "Oh, it's you." Even then I'm not sure as to what clicks anymore. The residents of the Center each have such diverse personalities because of the disease and each at a different stage of life (age) and stage of the disease itself. You can interact each time you go there by saying the same thing to the same ones because they don't change except I have noticed a decline in Craig and also that he sleeps more. You have to wake him...he's resting for his final journey home. Mike took him to church on Sunday and he didn't navigate a turn and fell. Mike said he panicked when he couldn't get Craig into the car. He was amazed that he couldn't talk him through it. He said it seemed like an eternity before he got him in. He's a psychologist and it made him anxious and he panicked and was glad to have him back at the center. That was Craig's last Sunday at going to church. I also think it is hard for him to leave the surroundings of the Center. He is very unsure of his footing and walks very slow and to go through a doorframe just throws him. I remember our doorframes at home. He would constantly ask when Steve was going to come and fix them. He would always bump his elbows. He does not know how to open a door or do the most ordinary of tasks. He sometimes stares or talks sideways before he realizes you are in front of him or vice versa. He is still very kind and gentle. He doesn't remember most names and yet can come up with something that I wouldn't remember. I talked to Rebecca tonight. She didn't know that Craig was in a care facility full time. He doesn't get up and walk or wander and he doesn't appear to be moody except sometimes he will cry or be teary eyed and I won't know what he is thinking about and it breaks your heart. He does talk about church. They do take the sacrament to them on Sunday afternoons. They had a youth group visit last night (Sunday) and adopt a grandparent program. I'm sure they didn't realize what they were up against. It makes you want to get out and start shouting about this disease. In fact, November is Alzheimer's month. Perhaps this is a good time to make people aware of the disease. I'll write a letter to the editor of our daily paper.

November 18, 1998. *"We wouldn't choose our trials, but hopefully we learn and become richer and more loving because of them"* — They rotate people for showers. Craig is pretty easy and doesn't mind being showered and is cooperative so he's one that is done early morning before breakfast and then they let him lie back down or sit him on the sofa. This morning at 5:30 they called to tell me they thought he was having seizures as he fell in the shower. It broke my heart to think of him falling down onto a tile floor. My heart aches and I knew this would come. (In August I had a struggle bathing and showering him and was frightened.) I went right down and he cried when he saw me. It reminded me of a little child being brave until his mom appears and then he could break down and cry. I spent the morning with him and went to work in the afternoon. Bill was there with him when I went back in the afternoon.

November 20, 1998. *"Be fully alert to whatever it is you are experiencing – learn and understand – feel and become"* — Today was even a harder day. He couldn't feed himself at all. We had to feed him. He's changing so much each day. His nights are harder too. He's not sleeping as well and tries to get up, doesn't know how and falls down. The beds are twin size and we put a mattress to the side after we get him to bed in case he falls out. He's like dead weight to try and get up because he doesn't know how to help at all. I stay longer each night. He fell twice within an hour tonight. He is so unsteady. I left about 2:00 a.m. and cried all the way home.

November 21, 1998. *"We each write our obituary each day by the way we live"* — Pretty much the same as yesterday. I stayed all night tonight. I sleep on the mattress beside him on the floor. You want to just hold him in your arms like a little baby – as truly his spirit body is.

November 26, 1998. *"Demands on our soul brings forth choice blessings"* — Thanksgiving Day – I know this will be our last Thanksgiving together. I fed Craig at the Center and then Steve came and we put Craig in the car and spent his last Thanksgiving together at their home with Steve, Wendy and the girls. We decided that Steve and Wendy would do Thanksgiving and Suzanne and Stephen would do Christmas. It was wonderful and sad and everything in between. It is so hard to see this once vital, energetic, bright, young person deteriorate before your eyes each day. Suzanne, Steve and their children stopped by the Center to visit. We don't say anything about special days just in case he has a flicker of memory. I think there is still something there at times or I wouldn't see his tears.

November 29, 1998. *"Every spirit builds itself a house, and beyond its house a world, and beyond its world a heaven. Know then that world exists for you."* – Ralph Waldo Emerson — He tried to sit down on one of the couches and missed it. He hit the back of his head and cried. He no longer calls himself dumb when he falls. We gave him an Ativan (1-mg) to relax him.

November 30, 1998. *"Each of our lives are beautifully woven together"* — He's falling more and more. He fell off the chair in the dining room. They put an apron on him and tie it around the chair to hold him there. Everyone is very innovative and we all do whatever it takes to have it all be "normal."

December 1, 1998. *"We should learn to celebrate death as we celebrate birth"* — He seems to be more anxious and cries a lot. He says he's scared. I remind him there is nothing to be frightened about and rub his neck and head to try and relax him. I now whisper in his ear about going home. I tell him it's okay if he wants to go home to Heavenly Father. And, that

Heavenly Father is ready for him when he wants to go. I've not been able to do that until now.

December 2, 1998. *"Find inner peace"* — The Center called me at work today. He fell and cut his head and wrist. They put bandages on him and gave him a Tylenol. He started to cry when he saw me walking in. He's childlike and appears brave until he sees me and then he breaks down and I sooth him as best I can wanting to cry myself. It tears me apart and breaks my heart. Norm and Tricia visited him today. Craig remembers Norm – not his name. He smiles and must have a flickering of the trips we took together. Norm jokes and laughs with him.

December 3, 1998. *"Your character is your destiny"* — I took some Orajel to him today and rubbed the inside of his mouth and gums. It looks like he's biting the inside of his cheeks. When Bill visited him today he couldn't believe the decline in Craig. Bill was as surprised as I was at the turn-around from the morning hours of sitting, non-coherent, staring and not 'there' at all. We put him in a wheelchair and walked him down to his room to see Steve's bear and pictures of the children. I'm sure he shed tears as he left like I always do. It's tough duty.

December 4, 1998. *"When your eulogy is being read – will you be happy with your life's actions"* — I spent the day at the Center. They called me early morning (3:00 a.m.) to tell me they thought he had seizured. I had him in a wheelchair today. He couldn't walk by himself. I wheeled him from the dining room table after breakfast to visit with Bob, Richard and Ed. Craig's spirits were good and we all fought back tears. We each know we are saying our good-byes. Bill stopped by again. He brought Craig fruit as he always does, but today he had a harder time figuring out how to eat it. He had to cut it into tiny pieces and help him eat it. It breaks your heart to see him deteriorate.

December 9, 1998. *"Get involved – reach out to others"* — They moved his bed against the wall and put his roommate in another room. I'm spending more nights. Pat and Tricia called again tonight to encourage me along. They visited Craig today and were shocked to see the decline since the last week they were there.

December 12, 1998. *"Heaven or hell is determined by the way we live our lives in the present"* — I spent all day at the Center. I love Saturdays and Sundays when I go early morning and stay until he is asleep. He's very constipated again. We're giving him prune juice and hope it helps. As their body and mind goes, they no long know how to have a bowel movement by themselves very easily. It is amazing the little things our bodies do that we so take for granted.

December 18, 1998. *"Act like a guardian angel"* — Today was our 33rd wedding anniversary. I stayed close to Craig today. He didn't move from the couch much and I just sat next to him rubbing his head and heck telling him how wonderful he was and how much he was loved. I hope he felt that love. How lucky I am that he is my eternal companion. I love you Hon. (Each night of our married life when we went to bed we would take turns saying, 'I love you Hon' and the other one responding back.) I still do it each night.

December 19, 1998. *"Our todays depend on our yesterdays and our tomorrows depend on our todays"* — They had a Christmas party at the Center. Suzanne and the children stopped by. Santa Claus came and gave each resident two gifts. I wrapped Craig up a new pair of sweat pants and pajama bottoms. They are the only things he wears now because they are the easiest to put on him and they are comfortable. He had no idea of what was happening around him. We had cookies and punch and he liked that. He seemed very tired. He went to bed at 9:00 and went right to sleep. I'll be glad when the holidays are over.

December 21, 1998. *"If you love yourself, forgive yourself, have compassion and understanding, then you will be able to give these gifts to others"* — He's very agitated today and seems upset. It took until about 11:00 to settle him down. He did okay with lunch. He was agitated again at bedtime. He woke up several times in the night yelling. You didn't know what he was saying just that he was upset.

December 24, 1998. *Our purpose in life is growth"* — We had Christmas dinner at Suzanne's. The aides helped me get him in the car and Suzanne and Stephen helped me get him out of the car and into their home. He had a hard time sitting at their table and it was so much like old times that it was hard to watch him. I had to feed him. He didn't know how to turn around in his chair and face the table. It was important to have that last time together just as we did at Thanksgiving at Steve and Wendy's. Memories ~ memories. They are what we cling to and really all we have when our loved ones go. But, how wonderful that we can imagine and remember the days gone by. We got him back into the car and I assured them the aides would help me back at the Center. When we got to the Center I thought I could make it with him to the gate and get help. I was totally wrong. I couldn't get him out of the car by myself and when I finally did he fell on the ice and while he laid there in the parking lot I had to unlock the gate, go yell for help and have two aides that were preparing other residents for bed come and help me. It was frightening to me. What heartache. We got him into bed and I not only cried all the way home, I cried myself to sleep.

December 25, 1998. *"Life is colored by our memories"* — I visited each of the children before I went to the Center this morning. I wanted this gift giving Christmas to be a gift they could remember because it would be the last gift from their father and grandfather. I gave each family a set of fun Christmas dishes that even had the plate and mug for Santa cookies and milk. I gave each of the children Christmas aprons and cookie kits so that each Christmas they could use them and remember the fun of making cookies at Christmas time and how much fun they had with Grandpa. I think I made it memorable for them. It was for me. I stayed late making the most of the time of this special day. The children visited him and I knew it was hard. We each realize this was our last Christmas together as a family as we have known it. But, again what wonderful memories we have. We are truly blessed.

December 26, 1998. *"To everything there is a season, a time to every purpose under the heaven: a time to be born, and a time to die..." (Ecclesiastes 3:1-2)* — Craig slept until 9:00. We didn't wake him for breakfast. He had breakfast and a snack then went back to sleep without lunch. He slept most of the day. I believe he's preparing for his journey home. I have so many mixed feelings inside of me now that I know his "graduation" day is fast approaching.

December 27, 1998. *"And whatsoever ye shall ask the Father in my name, which is right believing that ye shall receive, behold it shall be given unto you" (3 Nephi 18:20)* — He's very agitated today and extremely off balance. It is more than the usual leaning. He won't stay sitting down. He wants to move. I encourage him to sit and rub his head and shoulders to relax him. He had a very hard time going to the bathroom. It was a long day. He let us put him to bed early and I just knelt to the side of him, talked and rubbed his head. I cried all the way home.

December 28, 1998. *"Death comes to each of us"* — Today he's crying, yelling and a little bit of everything from time to time. We gave him a Tylenol when he said he had a headache. I spent the majority of the day just sitting on the couch by him holding his hand. (One of the female residents always likes to hold Craig's hand. He always thought she was a guy and would never let her hold his hand. When I hold his hand she said I wish I could do that because he is the most handsome guy here – you know that he's my boyfriend don't you. I assured her that I did and I'll only stay a minute. She would always try to hold his hand and he would fold his arms and say, 'don't touch'.) How wonderful that they touch each other and hold hands. Human touch is something that nothing can be replaced by. I will so miss being able to hold him as I sit close by his side rubbing his neck and stroking his head. I sometimes wonder who it is comforting. I actually know the answer. It's me. I do have my memories and how sweet they are.

December 29, 1998. *"God has a perfect plan to touch the lives of others through the lives of you and me"* — We're going to try and do more prune juice for him. It amazes me that people here that could be his father are more 'together' than he is. It's truly an unbelievable disease. He's off-balance and fallen five times today. We let him sleep on the couch tonight. It was easier than trying to move him. He woke up at 5:00 a.m. and wouldn't let anyone give him a pill to try to calm him. These days of agitation are hard days. They break my heart.

December 30, 1998. *"The city of happiness is found in the state of mind"* — It was another hard day. He wouldn't sleep tonight. He stayed on the couch again and it was about 4:00 a.m. before he went to sleep. In the early days at the Center I was always amazed at how the residents would walk around half the night and always appreciative that Craig would go to bed and stay there (most of the time). It's hard when they don't want to go to bed. You just know that sleep would make everything okay. Of course, it only makes everything okay in our world. And, they are not in 'our' world any longer. They are as little children.

December 31, 1998. *"I will do more than live – I will grow"* — He keeps trying to get up from the couch by himself and falls. As we were getting ready for dinner at 4:00 the power went out. Craig got very upset. He didn't like not being able to see or move. They handed out a lot of flash flights but it didn't help much and I didn't want to take Craig to bed yet. He didn't go to sleep until 4:00 a.m. yesterday. He's very repetitious and anxious. Mike and Linda stopped by to visit and invited me to dinner and a movie. This would be my last New Year's Eve with Craig and I wanted to stay and spend 'our' last one together. I wouldn't have left him no matter what. I have a lifetime of New Year's Eves, dinners and movies, and only this one last New Year's with my husband and the love of my life. He has certainly left a legacy of love.

January 1, 1999. *"The end is the beginning – if only we knew at the beginning what we know at the end"* — New Year's Day. Craig fell three times between 6:00 and 7:00 this morning. We gave him two Tylenols. He seemed wide-awake and was talking to someone. He seems calm and in good spirits. His speech is slurry and he seems to be talking to himself. He's very calm. Jan and Richard visited him. Stephen/Suzanne, Alex, Emily and Jamison visited. Steve/Wendy, Taylor and Madison also visited today. He would just sit and stare or sleep. There was very little interaction later in the day. It was hard on everyone. Pat, Kent and Tricia came at the end of the day. So, this is the beginning of the end. We've all bid the old year farewell. This is what we have been praying for and it's fast approaching. My heart aches. I already miss my one true love and he hasn't left me yet or at least his physical body. New Year's will never be the same.

January 2, 1999. *"Have courage for the great sorrows of life and patience for the small ones; and when you have accomplished your daily task, go to sleep in peace – God is awake"* — We started on stool softener pills this morning as well as everything else. Maybe something will help him. I can only hope and pray. Bill stopped by and brought me lunch. He has been such a good friend and supporter through this. He went home and called some of Craig's golfing buddies. He brought them back to see Craig. They, too, had not wanted to see Craig in his present surroundings. We all had some laughs. Craig appeared to have recognized them and laughed. Bill and I were both so surprised because Craig that morning knew nothing. It was like he would rally one last time. I think it was because of this that people didn't quite believe me at times about his decline. I truly believe people have to be told and made to believe so that we can all work together at getting this disease out and recognized.

January 3, 1999. *"Life is my journey, God is my guide and faith is my companion"* — He's having a harder time swallowing. I feed him only soft food. We dissolve the meds. He says his throat hurts. I don't know if the throat starts to close off as they forget how to swallow. It's heartbreaking. Bob and Richard visited today. We took a lot of pictures. We all sat by Craig and we each cried. I think the best way to describe him today was dazed. He would sit and not move, sleep and stare. I love you my Mr. Craig.

January 5, 1999. *"Trust in the Lord with all thine heart and lean not unto thine own understanding. In all thy ways acknowledge him and he shall direct thy paths" (Proverbs 3:5-6)* — Swallowing is still hard and he says it hurts. Maybe this is when the lungs start to fill and there starts to be some pressure. I don't know. A mysterious disease. I hope more research is done soon. Each of us knows the end is coming. The aides are so sweet and kind to him. They are kind and good to everyone. That is why I like this place so much. It has been like a family and a home for Craig and for myself.

January 6, 1999. *"Eternity is now – now is the time and this is the place"* — A so-so day. He was cold and clammy when we put him to bed tonight. The days and nights are getting harder. As much of an honor as it is to serve Craig it literally tears me apart inside and breaks my heart. I mostly sleep on the couch now days. I remember in the early days of caring for him and I would pray that he could shut his eyes and not wake up so he wouldn't have to suffer and that we who loved him so very much wouldn't have to watch his decline. I realize what a privilege it was to assist him and how few are blessed with the opportunity to serve the person they love the most as they prepare for their re-birth – death.

January 7, 1999. *"Come unto me, all ye that labour and are heavy laden, and I will give you rest. Take my yoke upon you, and learn of me; for I am meek and lowly in heart; and ye shall find rest unto your souls. For my yoke is easy, and my burden is light" (Matthew 11:28-30)* — One of the residents died today. She was probably in her 80's. She was actually more coherent and talked better than Craig. Craig has not been able to read from the beginning of his diagnosis in the fall of 1996. I was always amazed when one of the older residents who is over 80 years old would read a sign on the door. I've come to realize what matters most is to understand who we are and what we are doing here and have an absolute determination to return home to our Heavenly Father. This is a time of testing and at times seems to overshadow almost everything else. I resolve to do better each day.

January 8, 1999. *"Humble yourselves in the sight of the Lord, and he shall lift you up" (James 4:10)* — Craig slept through lunch today. He spit his sleeping pills out. He seemed to choke, even on the water. He doesn't know how to swallow very well anymore. He does better with liquids drawn up into a straw and just let it slide down his throat without really having to swallow, gulp or suck.

January 11, 1999. *"The Lord bless thee, and keep thee; the Lord make his face shine upon thee, and be gracious unto thee; the Lord lift up his countenance upon thee, and give thee peace" (Numbers 6:24-26)* — He fell several times today. It's getting harder and harder to watch the decline each day. I whispered in his ear again today that it's okay – he can go if he's ready that Heavenly Father is waiting. I then cried all the way home realizing how fast it is coming.

January 13, 1999. *"Therefore hold up your light that it may shine unto the world..." (3 Nephi 18:24)* — I'm having a harder time coming home and writing. I know I need to do this now, but it's hard. I did it in the beginning as a therapist to listen to me talk and now I do it as documentation to possibly help someone and perhaps that someone has only been me. I

January 14, 1999. *"No one lives without loss; it is part of life"* — His poor little back is so bruised from all of his falls. It breaks your heart to know that you can't help him. Collins' visited him today. They have been true friends. I know it isn't easy to visit him there. But, The Alzheimer Center is his home.

January 16, 1999. *"Beautiful memories last forever"* — The children visited him today. It gets harder to see the decline. When we walked him down to bed tonight he appeared to be dizzy, losing his balance and we had to hold him up. He slept well.

January 17, 1999. *"If we looked at mortality as the whole of existence, then pain, sorrow, failure, and short life would be calamity. But if we look upon life as an eternal thing stretching far into the pre-mortal past and on into the eternal post-death future, then all happenings may be put in proper perspective….Are we not exposed to temptations to test our strength, sickness that we might learn patience, death that we might be immortalized and glorified? If all the sick for whom we pray were healed, if all the righteous were protected and the wicked destroyed, the whole program of the Father would be annulled and the basic principle of the gospel, free agency, would be ended. No man would have to live by faith."* Spencer W. Kimball — I spent the day with Craig from early morning until bedtime. He was very agitated today. He never moved from the couch and the only liquids we could get down him was water drawn into a straw and let it drip down his throat otherwise he seemed to gag. His eyes were wild and dazed. I think I knew today that these days were ending and that Craig was gone. He slept off and on and I was ever so grateful when he was sleeping and seemed at peace. I will miss being able to touch him. He truly has been and is the love of my life. I am so grateful we are eternal companions. I cried all the way home and prayed to our Heavenly Father that he could be released from this earthly life. It was getting harder every day to see him slip away. Stephen had usually given him blessings of comfort but tonight he needed a blessing that he could be released. I called our neighbor when I got home from the Center and asked him if he would please give Craig a blessing. Craig deserved to be released from this earthly life and return home to his Heavenly Father. He ran a great race and deserved to go home. I will miss taking care of him.

January 18, 1999. *"I have fought a good fight, I have finished my course, I have kept the faith: Henceforth there is laid up for me a crown of righteousness, which the Lord, the righteous judge, shall give me at that day: and not to me only, but unto all them also that love his appearing." (2 Timothy 4:7-8)* — I spent the day at the Center with Craig. He appeared to be struggling and was unsteady. He went to bed fairly early tonight. It took three of us to get him down into bed. We left him in his sweats because his diapers were dry. We got him situated into bed and I kneeled down by his bed to rub his head and say a prayer with him. He kept telling me how much he loved me "Judy, I love you more than anything in the world ~ more than anything in the whole world" and he kept repeating this several times and I would keep telling him that I too loved him more than anything in the world but it was late and we should go to sleep. Craig knew me that night and I believe wanted to instill it in my mind and in my heart that before he left to return home I was loved and to remember it always. I know and I always will. What a memorable evening that was. I didn't realize then but these would be the last words he would speak except a few mutterings. I feel so loved and so very blessed for the wonderful times we had. I cried all the way home and thanked my Heavenly Father for this wonderful person I was so blessed to be loved by and married to – my best friend. I am so very grateful.

January 19, 1999. *"The Lord is my strength and my shield; my heart trusted in him and I am helped; therefore my heart greatly rejoiceth; and with my song will I praise him" (Psalms 28:7)* — At 4:00 a.m. they found him on the floor by the closet. He was crying. They called me and I got dressed and went right down. They took him to the dayroom on the couch and he slept there until mid-morning. His color doesn't seem the same. Around noon he was on the floor and had fallen off the couch again. Red would empty two sleeping capsules into sherbet and we would spoon that down him. He appears to be in a lot of pain. He is totally out of his mind today. I think his kidneys are starting to shut down now that he no longer knows how to eat or drink. His eyes almost look wild. I called the children and they called others. We all stayed with him today. Marcia called and Craig received Hospice (finally). They sent a hospital bed and a bottle of liquid Morphine for the pain he appears to be in. We got him into bed and put a hospital gown on him. We changed the diaper even though it wasn't wet. We cleaned him up. They left his other bed in the room by the hospital bed and that is where I slept (or laid). If he even wiggled I would give him a dropper of Morphine. I was nervous at first about being the one to administer the Morphine but Suzanne and the nurse assured me that I couldn't overdose him. I knew that he was now gone mentally and physically and I was not going to allow him to be in any pain. I watched him very closely. I played CD's softly believing your hearing is the last sense to go. His favorite was always, "Because I Have Been Given Much – I, too must give" and "Let There Be Peace On Earth" ~ my own favorite "An Angel Amongst Us" ~ that angel being Craig. We listened to those a lot that night. I talked to him a lot and as strange as it seems there was a peace in seeing him so at peace.

January 20, 1999. *"He that doeth the works of righteousness shall receive his reward, even peace in this world, and eternal life in the world to come." (D&C 59:23)* — I slept there and went home and changed quickly and returned. The children and Craig's family came off and on today. Craig is definitely resting up for his journey home. I keep eye drops in his eyes to lubricate them and keep a wet cloth over them to keep his eyelids closed. We have all prayed for this time to come and now it is here and you have many mixed feelings. I am trying to cherish the moments knowing these are the last of my Craig moments for the rest of our earthly life.

January 21, 1999. *"Well done thou good and faithful servant"* — Graduation Day. The best part of a journey is returning home. Craig completed his journey and returned home to his Heavenly Father at 6:40 p.m. I'm sure there was a glorious reunion by all those awaiting him on the other side. What was wonderful was we were all there. Bob and Richard stopped by to visit. They saw him in the morning. It was so very peaceful. Steve was teasing Craig about wanting to be free of volunteering and running free in Heaven. We all talked to him as though he was totally aware of us and perhaps he was. His lungs filled up those last hours of his life. Steve said the last prayer and not long afterwards Craig struggled for the last breath and we all delighted in that he was free and we were all so very proud of him and the valiant struggle he fought. He ran the race and crossed the finish line. I called Richard and he came after to say goodbye. Dave came to visit and did not know until he came into the room. He was stunned. Marsha and two of the aides helped clean him up and put some clothes on him for his van ride to the mortuary. As I cared for Craig those last two days I had trimmed his hair, rubbed his feet, clipped his nails the hair in his nose and ears that he was always so particular about. He even had a little blister on his foot that I couldn't figure out how he got it. I always rubbed his feet with lotion and kept his nails clipped since he was only able to shower and not bathe and soak his feet. Craig will be buried in his temple clothes with a few exceptions: his Nike running hat on his head and his bright colored Nike racing flats on his feet and we'll have the casket open all the way. He always said, 'running is my life.' I'm sure it will put people at ease — this is a good thing. It should make his friends smile to see him with his running shoes on — running all around Heaven. Craig deserved to go home and though we will miss him tremendously we know this is the best and how wonderful it is that Heavenly Father saw fit to allow him to go home to be with those that went before to prepare the way. Craig can now watch us and guide us as we move into a new phase of life until we are reunited again. This was a peaceful day.

January 22, 1999. *"…And blessed are all the pure in heart, for they shall see God." (3 Nephi 12:8)* — The children and I met to plan and prepare for the funeral and write the obituary. I had thought through some of these things because I truly believed we were going to lose Craig in December when he declined so rapidly. We each decided that we wanted to pay tributes to the person we all loved so very much. And, we knew him best. We also knew that Craig would want everything simple without a lot of fuss. Craig was a shy and quiet person never wanting a lot of attention paid to himself. We wanted his final tribute to be one that he would appreciate. We decided to have a picture of him running on the front of the program to honor him since running was his life and this was a tribute to that life. We knew his desires and would honor them.

January 26, 1999. *"That we may lead a quiet and peaceful life in all godliness and honesty" (1 Timothy 1:2)* — A Monday. We had a viewing to reminisce about his life. We had videos, pictures and some other memorabilia that showed Craig throughout his life as the bright, energetic, athletic person he was. I went to the mortuary early as they were bringing him up in the elevator so I could spend some time alone with him and talk. I put a wedding band on his hand and told him we were married again. He always loved wearing his wedding ring and when he was at the Alzheimer's Center I kept it at home. Actually, I wear it on a chain and bought him a new band to be buried with. We had friends and family come at the mortuary from 6-8. People started to come at 5:30 and didn't stop until after 9:00. They would remind us of the length of the line outside waiting and we seemed to rush people. I hope that people didn't sense any of that. There truly was an out-pouring of love for this tender, kind man. He truly led a quiet, peaceful life in godliness and honesty. What a wonderful tribute to Craig. We all love you Hon.

January 27, 1999. *"Peace I leave with you my peace I give unto you; not as the world giveth, give I unto you. Let not your heart be troubled, neither let it be afraid." (John 14:27)* — A Tuesday. We had a wonderful Celebration of Craig's Life (funeral). We held it at our church and it was filled. Steve and Suzanne each paid a wonderful tribute to their father and I, too, paid a tribute to Craig and let people know and understand a little about the disease as we went along our journey with Big Al. We played all of his favorite songs: Because I have Been Given Much, An Angel Amongst Us, piano solo, Joy, and at the conclusion of the dedication of the grave at Provo City Cemetery we played "Let There Be Peace on Earth – And, let it begin with me" — it was beautiful and a beautiful ending. It was a very snowy day today. It was almost fitting because Craig loved to run in the snow and today he was running free. Each of the grandchildren placed a stem of silk lilacs on the coffin. He loved the smell of lilacs in the spring. I'm sure Craig was embarrassed by the crowds and also honored to think his children paid such beautiful tributes to him. I'm sure he was proud. I know I was.

This is not the end………..Craig is still with us in spirit. He is in our memories and how wonderful those memories are.

ABOUT THE AUTHOR

Judy Seegmiller resides in Utah near her children and grandchildren. She is actively involved in reaching out to other Caregivers. She speaks to gerontology and social work classes to help them understand not only about the disease but also about the needs of the Caregiver. She volunteers her time in helping other caregivers understand their needs and to find humor and joy in being a Caregiver. She has donated some of her books to Adult Foster Care programs, caregivers, medical facilities, etc. in the hopes that they might find something useful in their journey of helping someone.

If you wish to contact the author, order a book, etc., you may do so by sending to:

BIG AL
P.O. Box 50212
Provo, UT 84605-0212